Anesthesiology Resident Manual
of Procedures

Claire Sampankanpanich Soria
Daniel E. Lee • Gerard R. Manecke

Anesthesiology Resident Manual of Procedures

A Step-by-Step Guide

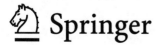

Claire Sampankanpanich Soria MD
Department of Anesthesiology
UCSD Medical Center
San Diego, CA
USA

Daniel E. Lee MD, PhD
Department of Anesthesiology
UCSD Medical Center
San Diego, CA
USA

Gerard R. Manecke MD
Department of Anesthesiology
UCSD Medical Center
San Diego, CA
USA

ISBN 978-3-030-65734-5   ISBN 978-3-030-65732-1   (eBook)
https://doi.org/10.1007/978-3-030-65732-1

This Springer imprint is published by the registered company Springer Nature Switzerland AG
The registered company address is: Gewerbestrasse 11, 6330 Cham, Switzerland

Acknowledgments

The contents of this book are based on the outstanding education that I received as an anesthesiology resident while training at the University of California, San Diego. I must give special thanks to the many UCSD educators who have taught me over the years, including, but not limited to: Dr. Daniel E. Lee, Dr. Gerard R. Manecke, Dr. Ruth Waterman, Dr. Jonathan Benumof, Dr. Alyssa Brzenski, Dr. Piyush Patel, Dr. Rodney Gabriel, Dr. Arthur Lam, Dr. John Drummond, Dr. Lawrence Weinstein, Dr. Leon Chang, Dr. Karim Rafaat, Dr. Mark Greenberg, and Dr. Rick Bellars.

About the Book

This book was developed with the goal of helping medical trainees in all stages of training who work in critical care settings in the operating room, emergency department, and the intensive care unit. In such environments, we must provide quality medical care even under high stress situations with little time to prepare. The purpose of this book is to enable learners to quickly prepare for critical procedures and perform them well.

Contents

About the Author

Claire Sampankanpanich Soria is a board-certified pediatric anesthesiologist. She completed her undergraduate training at the University of California, Los Angeles; medical school at Johns Hopkins University School of Medicine; residency in anesthesiology at the University of California, San Diego; and fellowship in pediatric anesthesiology at Children's Hospital of Los Angeles. She currently works on faculty at the University of California, San Diego.

Airway Anatomy and Tracheobronchial Tree

Preoperative Airway Evaluation

Ideally patient is sitting upright at 90° angle to optimize view of the mouth [1].

1. Long upper incisors
2. Overriding upper incisors ('buck teeth')
3. Mandibular prognathism (ability to move mandibular incisors in front of maxillary incisors)
4. Inter-incisor distance
   (a) >3 cm to fit laryngoscope blade into mouth
   (b) Normal mouth opening = 5–6 cm
   (c) Flange of Mac and Miller blades = 2 cm
5. Oropharyngeal classification (distance from tongue base to roof of mouth)
   (a) Mallampati I: can see soft palate, tonsillar pillars, tip of uvula, fauces on either side of uvula
   (b) Mallampati II: loss of the tonsils; still can see uvula and fauces on either side of the uvula
   (c) Mallampati III: loss of tip of uvula and the fauces; can only see the base of uvula
   (d) Mallampati IV: loss of the base of the uvula
6. Rule out narrow high-arched palate (oropharyngeal volume laterality)
7. Mandibular space length = thyromental distance (TMD)
   (a) Ideally >3 fingerbreadths or 6 cm
8. Mandibular space compliance
9. Length of neck
10. Thickness of neck
11. Range of motion of head and neck

© The Author(s), under exclusive license to Springer Nature Switzerland AG 2021
C. Sampankanpanich Soria et al., *Anesthesiology Resident Manual of Procedures*,
https://doi.org/10.1007/978-3-030-65732-1_1

Tracheobronchial Tree Anatomy

Identifying Carina (Fig. 1.1)
- Look for the right upper lobe takeoff. False. Can still be fooled.
- Look for the left mainstem bronchus.
  - Other than the trachea itself, only the left mainstem bronchus will look long and straight.
  - Left mainstem bronchus will have at least 8–10 cartilaginous rings, ~5 cm long.
  - The bronchus intermedius, by contrast, will be shorter.

Importance of Knowing Subsegmental Bronchi
- To estimate loss of ventilation from lobectomy
- E.g., after left lower lobe resection, loss of 5 subsegmental bronchi, or $5/10 = 50\%$ of left lung, and $5/20 = 25\%$ of whole lung is observed

Distances to Know

Teeth to vocal cords = 15 cm [1]
   Nose to vocal cords = 18 cm (from nose, add 3 cm due to curvature of nasopharynx)

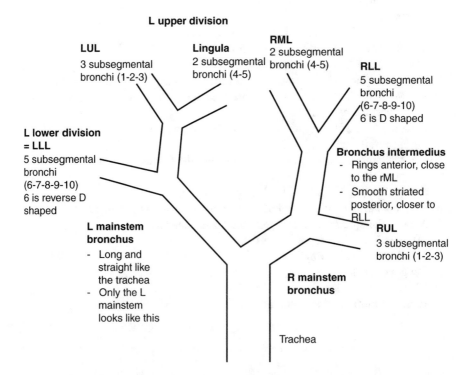

Fig. 1.1   Illustration of tracheo-bronchial tree anatomy including number of subsegments

Teeth to the top of epiglottis = 12 cm
Nose to the top of epiglottis = 15 cm
Top of epiglottis to vocal cords = 3 cm
Trachea length = ~12–15 cm (±1 cm for every ±1" from height of 5'7")
Yellow oral airway = ~9 cm (terminates ~3 cm from the top of epiglottis)
Pink oral airway = ~10 cm

Estimating the Depth of the Endotracheal Tube (ETT) for Intubation (Fig. 1.2)/(Table 1.1)

1. Gold standard: anesthesiologist visualizes the endotracheal tube (ETT) cuff going 1–2 cm past the vocal cords
2. Listening for breath sounds
   (a) Ideal: auscultate in the axilla; bilateral breath sounds
   (b) Can be fooled by transmitted breath sounds from right to left
   (c) Absence of breath sounds over the stomach
3. Predicted measurement (in a 7.0 ETT for a 5'7" adult)

Fig. 1.2 Illustration of the structure of the pharynx including the nasopharynx, oropharynx, and laryngopharynx

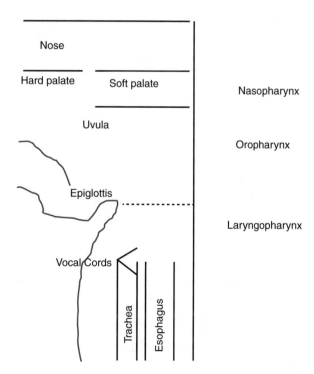

Table 1.1 Distances between pharyngeal landmarks and endotracheal tube

Teeth to the top of epiglottis	12 cm
Top of epiglottis to vocal cords	3 cm
Proximal end to distal end of cuff of ETT	3 cm
Distal end of cuff to tip of ETT	2 cm
+ cuff advanced 1–2 cm past vocal cords	1–2 cm
Depth of ETT at teeth	21–22 cm

Reference

1. Stone DJ, Gal TJ. Chapter 42: airway management. In: Miller RD, editor. Anesthesia. Philadelphia: Churchill Livingstone; 1994. p. 1404–19.

Optimizing Intubation Positioning

2

Goals of Ramp (Table 2.1)/(Table 2.2)
1. Tragus in line with sternum
2. Flat chest
3. Room to lift the chin up

Best place to double check ramp: stand lateral to patient and squat down to eye level with patient. Do this with every adjustment. Ask patient to tilt chin up and verify room for extension.

© The Author(s), under exclusive license to Springer Nature Switzerland AG 2021
C. Sampankanpanich Soria et al., *Anesthesiology Resident Manual of Procedures*,
https://doi.org/10.1007/978-3-030-65732-1_2

How to Make a Ramp

Table 2.1   Comparison of the pros and cons of common techniques used to make a ramp to optimize patient positioning for intubation

Equipment	Technique	Pros	Cons
Blankets	Stack of pancakes: 1 foam donut and 1 small towel under patient's head (standard). Add "x" number of blankets under head + "x" number of blankets under chest. Reassess, remove extra blankets as needed. Rolled hotdogs: 1 foam donut and 1 small towel under patient's head (standard). Add "x" number of blankets rolled into a thick roll, placed under shoulder blades horizontally.	Blankets are readily available in the OR, cheap, easy to use.	Usually will need to lift these after intubation so surgeons have a level operating field. Hard to find enough blankets outside of the OR.
Pillows	1 foam donut and 1 small towel under patient's head (standard). Add 1–2 pillows under the shoulder blades and lower half of neck horizontally.	Readily available outside the OR.	Soft, sagging, not as dense as blankets. Must lift patient to remove after intubation.
Pre-made ramp	Lay patient on pre-made ramp, usually foam.	Pre-made.	Not readily available Not one size fits all. Must lift patient to slide out after intubation; large, hard to remove.
OR table	Elevate head of bed using bed remote. Then use latch system to tilt down for head extension.	Don't need extra equipment. Don't need to lift patient to remove blankets/pillows.	Not every bed has the latch system (e.g., removed for urology cases, neurosurgery).

Common Pitfalls and How to Approach Them

Table 2.2 Common challenges to optimizing patient positioning for intubation, including performing intubations outside of the operating room such as in a gurney or intensive care unit bed

Scenario	Challenges	Techniques
Out of OR intubations	Coding patient Rushed, stressful environment, hard to focus Unfamiliar environment Different equipment Hospital beds: lumpy, covered with blankets/ food trays/cables, patients sagging low in bed ICU beds broken, fewer features to adjust positioning	Take deep breaths Assess and optimize intubation position while performing H&P and preparing equipment Time spent at beginning optimizing position = less time spent on multiple intubation attempts Rushing in non-ideal positioning = repeated unsuccessful intubations, wasted time, hypoxia, edematous and bloody airway Ask RNs and RTs for assistance Pull patient close to you Remove headboard Fold the handlebars down at head of bed Use pillows, rolled sheets/blankets for shoulder roll → limited supplies, may not have anything to place under occiput. Can ask RN/RT to hold patient's head in good sniff position for you if needed Elevate head of bed; if bed broken, use manual latch under the mattress or put in reverse Trendelenberg (caution with reverse T-berg: may exacerbate hypotension in already hypotensive, hypovolemic patients)
Intubating in a gurney or ICU bed in the OR	Done for patient comfort (orthopedic surgery patient, plan to flip prone for surgery, ortho table/ frame) Hesitant to reposition patient awake due to pain	Same as out of OR intubations (see above)
Morbidly obese patient	Patient may be in pain and refuse to position self on ramp Resistance from OR staff to move heavy patient, history of lift injuries Lack of availability of moving help or equipment	Give 25–50 mcg fentanyl early to minimize pain Psychological buy-in: reassure patient that the discomfort is temporary, will be asleep soon after pre-oxygenation Educate patient and staff that goal is to decrease the risk of difficult intubation Call for additional providers to help move patient Use bean bag or other assistive devices Reassure surgeons that ramp will be removed as soon as ETT is secured
Over-extension	Too many layers under the shoulder blades Neck over-extended, trachea too anterior	Stand lateral to patient, squat down, and double-check the 3 criteria for ideal positioning

(continued)

Table 2.2 (continued)

Scenario	Challenges	Techniques
Over-flexion	Too many layers under the head Pediatrics: large occiput resting on another foam donut cushion Thick hair, dreadlocks, weaves, wigs, buns	Prior to induction, ask patient to tilt chin up and verify adequate room for extension Pediatrics: once child is asleep, move the foam donut under neck and extend the head with right hand Hair: politely ask patient to push hair laterally or remove wig
Cervical spine precautions	Not allowed to extend neck even with cervical collar on	Depending on airway exam, may consider alternatives to direct laryngoscopy (glidescope, FOB) Can still elevate head of bed or tilt in reverse T-berg
Protuberant chest	Obese patient Breast implants Pregnant patient	Ensure enough layers underneath back to allow for head extension

How to Assemble and Use the Fiberoptic Scope and Tower

3

Range of Motion

1. Advance deeper.
2. Pull out.
3. Turn clockwise.
4. Turn counterclockwise.
5. Pull lever down → Flex scope anteriorly.
6. Push lever up → Flex scope posteriorly.

How to Maneuver the Scope

1. Apply lubricant to scope and equipment.
2. Apply antifog to scope tip.
3. Center image, then readvance scope.
4. Center, then advance. Center, then advance. Center then advance.
5. Slow movements.
6. Small movements.
7. Do not advance scope unless there is a clear image.
8. You do not get points for speed. You will just end up lost.
9. If secretions obscure the image, gently touch the tip of the scope to the tracheal wall to clear.
10. For shorter providers, use a stepstool.
11. Keep the scope long and straight so movements up top match movements down low.

© The Author(s), under exclusive license to Springer Nature Switzerland AG 2021
C. Sampankanpanich Soria et al., *Anesthesiology Resident Manual of Procedures*,
https://doi.org/10.1007/978-3-030-65732-1_3

Features on Standard Anesthesia Scopes

1. Suction port
    (a) Located on right side of handle.
    (b) Must connect standard suction tubing to suction adaptor connected to handle.
    (c) To spray fluids (e.g., topicalize airway with preservative-free lidocaine, spray normal saline to perform a bronchoalveolar lavage), must disconnect suction tubing and suction adaptor. Ideally use a slip tip syringe to prevent leakage of fluid around the port.
2. Button to activate suction
    (a) Located on anterior part of handle
    (b) Usually use index finger to press this button
3. Lever to retroflex or anteroflex the scope tip
    (a) Located on posterior part of handle
    (b) Usually use thumb to press down on and pull up on lever
4. Variations
    (a) Depends on institutional availability.
    (b) Handle may have an eyepiece attached to it.
        (i) Only the scope operator can see the airway.
    (c) Handle may have a small video screen attached to it.
        (i) Must repeatedly rotate the screen as scope is repositioned and reoriented.
    (d) Handle may be connected to separate video monitor.
        (i) Do not need to adjust a separate screen.
        (ii) Everyone can see the airway.
    (e) Additional features on scopes used by ENT and Pulmonary and Critical Care
        (i) Ports for biopsies
        (ii) Buttons to freeze images, record videos, and save imaging files
        (iii) Often have larger suction channels, better for clearing thick secretions

How to Hold the Scope

- Personal and institutional preference.
- Generally hold the navigation handle with the right hand, and use left hand to hold the scope itself.

Where to Stand Relative to the Patient

- Personal preference
- Only applicable to awake fiberoptic intubations
- Provider stands facing patient/head of bed
    - Improves face-to-face communication.

- Disorienting because image is reversed from traditional view.
- How to make scope orientation easier: hold the scope the same way ENT surgeons to. Continue to hold the scope in standard format, such that turning clockwise turns to *provider's* right; pushing lever down will flex scope anterior to *provider*. Right of screen is patient's left, but this becomes irrelevant. The target is still the trachea.
- Provider stands at head of bed, facing the feet
  - Standard position, traditional views of airway

How to Set up the Fiberoptic Scope (FOB) and Tower

1. Gather necessary equipment
   (a) Tower: includes monitor, box for light source, and box for video source.
   (b) Scope
       (i) Scope size depends on internal diameter of endotracheal tube, tracheostomy tube, and patient airway.
       (ii) Choose the largest scope that will fit into the airway/tube to minimize slippage. Gaps between scope and tube equals tube getting hung up soft tissues.
       (iii) 3.0, aka "pediatric" scope, aka "small" – smaller the scope, poorer the image resolution.
       (iv) 4.0, aka "medium."
       (v) 5.0, aka "large."
   (c) Suction tubing.
   (d) Nonsterile gauze or scratch pad to clean scope tip.
   (e) Antifog solution.
   (f) Lubricant for scopes – silicone. Do *not* use surgical jelly; counterproductive – will dry up around scope and ETT, causing them to stick together (Fig. 3.1)/(Fig. 3.2)/(Fig. 3.3).
   (g) Slip-tip syringe.
   (h) Preservative-free lidocaine.

Fig. 3.1 Choose the correct lubricant. Surgical jelly on the left is not ideal. Antifog solution is in the middle. On the right is the appropriate lubricant for the scope

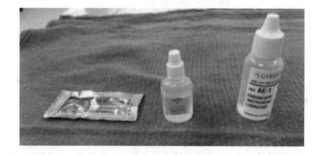

Fig. 3.2 Pulling the lever down will move the scope tip anteriorly (anteroflexion)

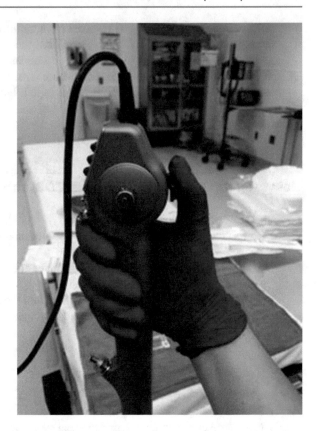

(i) Normal saline.
(j) PRN method of intubation.
    (i) Intubating oral airways (traditional pink and yellow vs. white Ovassapian) (Fig. 3.4)/(Fig. 3.5)
    (ii) Non-sterile gauze
    (iii) Cook LMA
    (iv) LMA Unique
    (v) Aintree catheter
    (vi) ETT exchanger
    (vii) Topicalization agents and equipment
        1. Preservative-free lidocaine
        2. Nebulizer
        3. Lidocaine ointment and tongue depressor
2. Plug in tower power cord to outlet.
  (a) Two large buttons for the video box and light box should turn on to an orange color (standby mode).
  (b) If the lights do not turn on, the tower may need to be restarted. Underneath the tower at the very bottom, close to the floor, there is a switch. Turn this switch off and on to reboot the tower.

Fig. 3.3 Pushing the lever up will move the scope tip posteriorly (posteroflex)

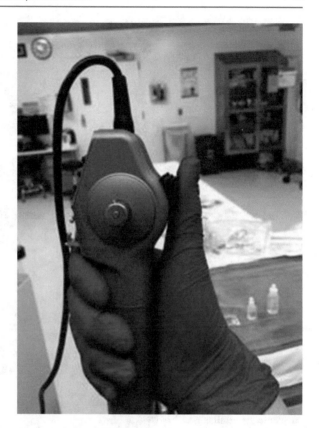

3. Press the buttons on the video box and light box to turn on. The button colors will change from orange to green.
4. Connect lightsource on scope to light box on tower.
   (a) The lightsource connection on the scope has a 2″ metal rod sticking out; this rod goes into the lightbox directly. The lightsource on the scope also has a faceplate with pins and yellow dots; this faces to the provider's right. Ensure that these align with the light box. A click will sound with proper placement.
   (b) Notice the brighten/darken spectrum buttons on the far right.
   (c) If the image is too bright, everything looks white.
   (d) If the image is too dark, everything looks black.
   (e) Common pitfall: the provider makes the light bulb too dark.
5. The lightbox defaults to standby. To turn on the bulb, click the power on button. To put in standby, click the standby button.
   (a) Common pitfall: provider forgets to turn on the light bulb by taking off of "standby."
6. Connect the video source on the scope to the video box on the tower.
   (a) The video box has a thick pigtail cord hanging out, with a faceplate with matching pins. This plate must align with the pins on the light source from the scope, which is now plugged into the light box on the tower.

Fig. 3.4 Intubating oral airways

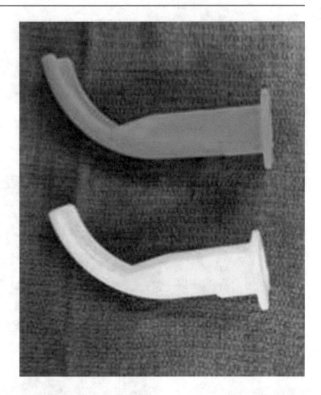

Fig. 3.5 Tape the 15 mm adaptor to the ventilator. Do not lose

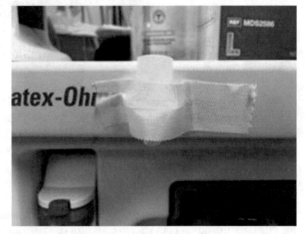

    (b) Once the yellow dots are aligned, push the plate in and rotate clockwise.

    (c) A click will sound when they are properly connected.

7. Coat (FOB) scope with lubricant. Run all airway equipment through the scope to ensure everything passes smoothly. A little lubricant goes a long way.

8. Proceed with intubation.

Asleep Fiberoptic Intubations

4

Method #1: Intubating Without Maintaining Ventilation, Using an Intubating Oral Airway

Equipment Needed
- Fiberoptic tower
- Appropriate-sized fiberoptic scope
- Appropriate-sized ETT
- Antisialogogue (normally glycopyrrolate)
- Induction agents of choice (usually propofol and rocuronium)
- Elbow adaptor compatible with bronchoscope
- Intubating oral airway (routinely pink 10 cm for men, yellow 9 cm for women; occasionally white Ovassapian)
- Lubricant
- Antifog solution

Steps
1. Set up FOB scope and tower. Lubricate all equipment and ensure everything slides smoothly over one another.
2. Remove the 15 mm adaptor from the endotracheal tube and place this in a secure location. (Usually taped to the ventilator or FOB tower.) (Fig. 3.5).
3. Pre-load the endotracheal tube onto the FOB scope. Secure to the scope handle using a strip of tape or a rubber band (Fig. 4.1)/(Fig. 4.2).
4. Administer glycopyrrolate at least 10–15 min prior to intubation.
   (a) Standard dose is 0.2 mg IV
   (b) Increase to 0.4 mg IV if lots of secretions
   (c) Consider holding or decreasing to 0.1 mg IV if underlying cardiac pathology that would be exacerbated by tachycardia

Fig. 4.1 A fiberoptic bronchoscope with an endotracheal tube taped to the base of the handle. The 15 mm adaptor has been removed from the endotracheal tube. This makes it easier to maneuver the scope during intubation

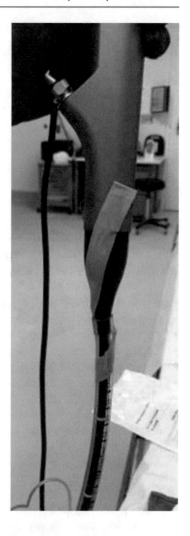

Fig. 4.2 A fiberoptic bronchoscope that has been pre-loaded with an endotracheal tube and an intubating oral airway

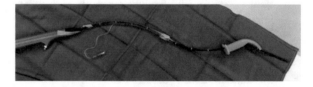

5. Position patient for intubation.
   (a) Even though the plan is to perform asleep fiberoptic intubation, position patient optimally (goals: flat chest, room for head extension, tragus in line with sternum).
   (b) Proper positioning will still improve view under FOB.
6. Standard pre-oxygenation.
7. Standard IV induction of patient.
8. Remove face mask.
9. Insert intubating oral airway.
10. If additional provider (OR RN, anesthesia tech, anesthesiologist) is available, ask them to apply jaw thrust to optimize view, maintain oral airway in position, and elevate soft tissue – this step can make a tremendous difference in view and ability to achieve bronchoscope entry into trachea.
11. Insert fiberoptic scope through the oral airway, advance past the tongue, and identify the vocal cords.
12. Advance scope past the vocal cords to 1–2 cm above the carina. Survey tracheobronchial tree if desired.
13. Ask assistant to undo the tape/rubber band and gently slide the ETT over scope and into the trachea.
14. If resistance is met, gently rotate the ETT counterclockwise. Likely it is hung up on the arytenoids posteriorly.
15. Slowly pull back the FOB scope while leaving the ETT in the trachea. Verify trachea and then ETT are visualized as scope is removed.
16. Slide the oral airway out of the mouth, over the ETT, being careful not to accidentally extubate the patient.
17. Reconnect the 15 mm adaptor to the ETT.
18. Connect ETT to ventilator circuit.
19. Test ventilate. Ensure adequate $ETCO_2$ and waveform.
20. Place patient on ventilator at programmed settings.
21. If desired, reinsert FOB scope to reconfirm positioning of ETT tip 1–2 above carina and survey tracheobronchial tree.

Method #2: Intubating Without Maintaining Ventilation, Without an Oral Airway

Equipment Needed
- Fiberoptic tower
- Appropriate-sized fiberoptic scope
- Appropriate-sized ETT
- Antisialogogue (normally glycopyrrolate)
- Induction agents of choice (usually propofol and rocuronium)

- Green elbow adaptor compatible with bronchoscope
- Lubricant
- Antifog solution
- Non-sterile gauze
- Second provider to assist

Steps
1. Set up FOB scope and tower. Lubricate all equipment and ensure everything slides smoothly over one another.
2. Pre-load the endotracheal tube with the 15 mm adaptor onto the FOB scope. Secure to the scope handle using a strip of tape or a rubber band.
3. Administer glycopyrrolate at least 10–15 min prior to intubation.
   (a) Standard dose is 0.2 mg IV.
   (b) Increase to 0.4 mg IV if lots secretions.
   (c) Consider holding or decreasing to 0.1 mg IV if underlying cardiac pathology that would be exacerbated by tachycardia.
4. Position patient for intubation.
   (a) Even though plan is to perform asleep fiberoptic intubation, position patient optimally (goals: flat chest, room for head extension, tragus in line with sternum).
   (b) Proper positioning will still improve view under FOB.
5. Standard pre-oxygenation.
6. Standard IV induction of patient.
7. Remove face mask.
8. Second provider uses gauze to hold distal part of half of patient's tongue and retract it outwards. If possible, also apply jaw thrust to elevate soft tissue – this step can make a tremendous difference in view and ability to achieve bronchoscope entry into trachea.
9. Insert fiberoptic scope directly into the oropharynx, advance past the tongue, and identify the vocal cords.
10. Advance scope past the vocal cords to 1–2 cm above the carina. Survey tracheobronchial tree if desired.
11. Ask assistant to undo the tape/rubber band and gently slide the ETT over scope and into the trachea.
12. If resistance is met, gently rotate the ETT counterclockwise. Likely it is hung up on the arytenoids.
13. Slowly pull back the FOB scope while leaving the ETT in the trachea. Verify trachea and then ETT are visualized as scope is removed.
14. Connect ETT to ventilator circuit.
15. Test ventilate. Ensure adequate $ETCO_2$ and waveform.
16. Place patient on ventilator at programmed settings.
17. If desired, reinsert FOB scope to reconfirm positioning of ETT tip 1–2 above carina and survey tracheobronchial tree.

Method #3: Intubating While Mask Ventilating, Using an Oral Airway and an Aintree Catheter

Equipment
- Aintree catheter (6.0, 19.0 Fr, 56 cm)
- 4.0 mm FOB scope (intermediate sized)
- 7.0 ETT
- Lubricant
- Antifog solution
- Pink or yellow intubating oral airway
- Face mask
- Black straps to hook onto face mask
- Elbow adaptor compatible with FOB scope
- Second provider to assist

Steps
1. Set up FOB scope and tower. Lubricate all equipment and ensure everything slides smoothly over one another.
2. Preload the Aintree catheter onto the FOB scope. Secure with a piece of tape.
3. Lubricate the 7.0 ETT with the 15 mm adaptor on. Set off to the side for now.
4. Position patient for intubation.
5. Standard pre-oxygenation with face mask already connected to bronch elbow adaptor.
6. Standard IV induction.
7. Insert the intubating oral airway midline.
   (a) Note that these have a tendency to pop out. Compared to the question mark (?) shape of a regular oral airway, these are completely curved.
8. Then, apply bilateral jaw thrust and push down on the oral airway with both thumbs to settle the oral airway into the oropharynx properly.
9. Maintain jaw thrust with your left hand as you use your right hand to put the face mask on the patient.
10. Once the face mask is secure, slip your left hand over the face mask and use your right hand to connect the black face mask straps on the right side of the face mask (Fig. 4.3).
11. Then hold jaw thrust with the right hand, and use your left hand to connect the straps to the left side of the face mask.
    (a) Ensure that at least one hand is always applying chin lift and jaw thrust.
    (b) If you completely release chin lift and jaw thrust, the oral airway will pop out.
12. Ensure adequate bag mask ventilation using $ETCO_2$ capnogram.
13. Switch to ventilator at programmed settings and ensure continued appropriate ventilation using $ETCO_2$ capnogram. Keep peak inspiratory pressures as low as possible to avoid filling stomach with gas.

Fig. 4.3 Illustration of equipment setup when intubating with a fiberoptic bronchoscope and Aintree catheter through a face mask and into an intubating oral airway

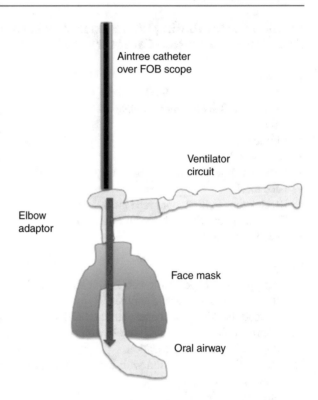

Aintree catheter over FOB scope

Ventilator circuit

Elbow adaptor

Face mask

Oral airway

14. Ask the second provider to stand at the right side of the patient, facing you.
15. Maintaining chin lift and jaw thrust, allow the second provider to take over managing the face mask.
16. Take the FOB scope that has been preloaded with the Aintree catheter.
17. Carefully advance the FOB scope into the elbow adaptor, through the face mask, and through the intubating oral airway (Fig. 4.4).
    (a) Watch with your eyes. Make sure you are not advancing the scope outside of the oral airway (e.g., into the patient's nose).
    (b) The oral airway may require some repositioning to maintain it midline.
18. Advance the scope past the tongue, identify the vocal cords, advance past the cords, and locate the carina.
19. Untape the Aintree catheter and gently slide the Aintree over the scope, to terminate 1–2 cm above the carina. Be careful not to mainstem the Aintree, as this will cause trauma to the airway.
20. Pull the FOB scope completely out of the oral airway, face mask, and bronch elbow. Be careful not to remove the Aintree.
21. Remove all equipment except the Aintree; remove the oral airway, face mask, and bronch elbow.
22. At this point, hold ventilation as the face mask is no longer on the patient.
23. Slide the ETT over the Aintree. Note the depth of the ETT.

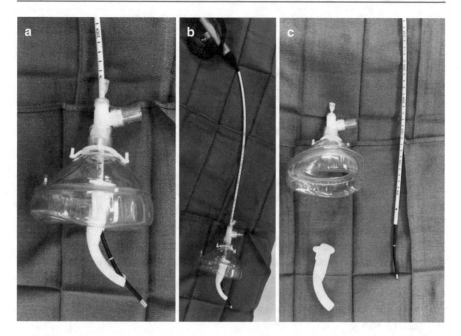

Fig. 4.4 (**a/b/c**) Aintree catheter preloaded over the fiberoptic scope, passing through an intubating oral airway, bronchoscopy elbow adaptor, and face mask

24. Remove the Aintree catheter.
25. Connect ETT to circuit and resume ventilation. Verify appropriate $ETCO_2$ capnogram.
26. Reconfirm position of ETT using FOB scope.

Method #4: Intubating While Ventilating Through an LMA, Using an ETT Exchanger

Equipment
- Intubating LMA
  - Cook LMA: works the best; wide tube to accommodate ETT and FOB scope; short tube length so when scope exists the bowl of LMA, superior enough to see the vocal cords versus so deep that exit directly into the esophagus
  - LMA Unique: wide tube, longer tube than Cook LMA, less curved; may need to cut the LMA tube to shorten it or use a longer ETT such as a nasal RAE or MLT (microlaryngoscopy tube).
- 5.0 mm FOB scope (large sized)
- 7.0 ETT
  - LMA Unique size 5 will fit a 7.0 ETT
  - LMA Unique size 4 will fit a 6.0 ETT

- ETT extender appropriately sized to push ETT through LMA after successful intubation.
  - If no ETT extender is available, use a 6.0 ETT. Tear off the pilot bulb and disconnect the 15 mm adaptor.
- Lubricant
- Antifog solution
- Face mask
- Elbow adaptor compatible with FOB scope

Steps
1. Set up FOB scope and tower. Lubricate all equipment and ensure everything slides smoothly over one another.
2. Remove 15 mm adaptor from ETT and tape to ventilator.
3. Set aside the FOB scope and ETT for now.
4. Position patient for intubation.
5. Standard pre-oxygenation with face mask already connected to bronch elbow adaptor.
6. Standard IV induction including paralytic. Do not want patient to cough and buck while using the FOB scope.
7. Insert LMA.
8. Disconnect cap on LMA (red or purple, hangs off to side).
9. Insert ETT directly into LMA. Do not advance past 18 cm. Just enough for ETT tip to exit the LMA bevel. If advance ETT is too deep, it may go into the esophagus (Fig. 4.5)/(Fig. 4.6)/(Fig. 4.7).
10. Connect bronch elbow adaptor to ETT. Hook up to ventilator circuit. Test ventilation by manually bagging. Verify appropriate $ETCO_2$ capnogram. Turn on ventilator (Fig. 4.8)/(Fig. 4.9).

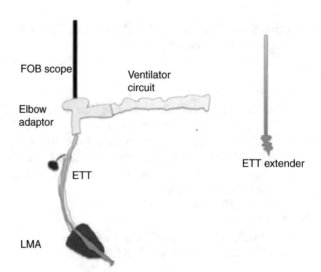

Fig. 4.5 Illustration of intubating with a fiberoptic bronchoscope loaded through an endotracheal tube that has been loaded into a laryngeal mask airway

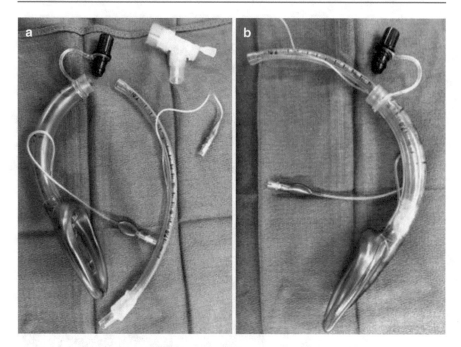

Fig. 4.6 (**a/b**) A 7.0 cuffed endotracheal tube loaded into a Cook laryngeal mask airway size 4.5 at a depth of 18 cm with the cap of the LMA removed

Fig. 4.7 View of the tip of the endotracheal tube positioned just proximal to the opening of the bowl of the laryngeal mask airway

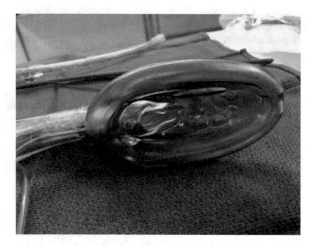

Fig. 4.8 An endotracheal tube loaded into a laryngeal mask airway, with a 90 degree angle bronchoscopy elbow adaptor connected to the endotracheal tube to enable continued ventilation through the ETT/LMA while the provider performs fiberoptic bronchoscopy through the ETT/LMA simultaneously

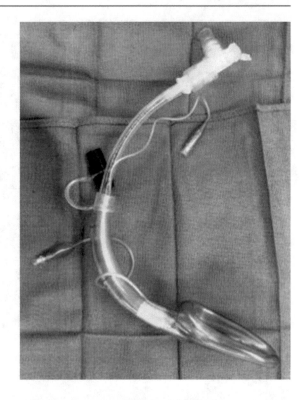

Fig. 4.9 A fiberoptic bronchoscope inserted through a bronchoscopy elbow adaptor into an endotracheal tube, which has been loaded into a laryngeal mask airway

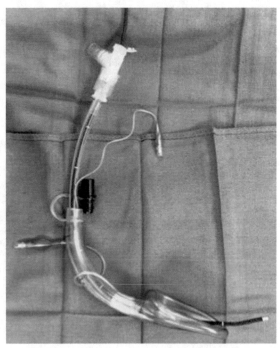

Fig. 4.10 The endotracheal tube has been advanced through the LMA and the fiberoptic bronchoscope and bronchoscopy elbow adaptor have been removed from the ETT/LMA setup

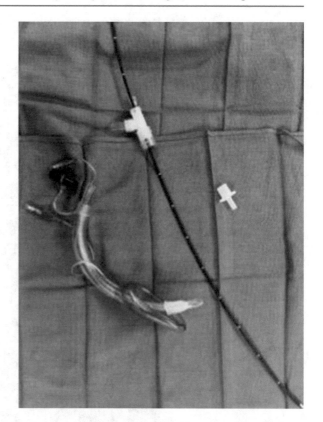

11. Ask second provider to hold up the circuit system so it does not fall to the side.
12. Take FOB scope and insert into the bronch elbow adaptor, into the ETT.
13. Advance FOB scope out of the ETT and LMA bowl. Likely will need to antero-flex to visualize the vocal cords. Advance past the vocal cords to the carina.
14. Slide the ETT into the LMA, over the FOB scope, until it hubs.
15. Remove the FOB scope.
16. Disconnect the elbow/circuit from the ETT (Fig. 4.10).
17. Insert the ETT extender into the proximal part of 7.0 ETT (Fig. 4.11)/(Fig. 4.12).
    (a) Of note, if an ETT extender is not available, a 6.0 endotracheal tube with the 15 mm adaptor removed can be used instead in the same fashion (Fig. 4.15)/(Fig. 4.16)/(Fig. 4.17)/(Fig. 4.18)/(Fig. 4.19).
18. Carefully remove the LMA by sliding it out over the 7.0 ETT and the ETT extender (Fig. 4.13).
19. Disconnect the ETT extender from the 7.0 ETT.
20. Connect the 15 mm adaptor to the 7.0 ETT (Fig. 4.14)/(Fig. 4.15).
21. Connect ETT to circuit and verify ventilation with ETCO$_2$ capnogram.
22. Reconfirm location of ETT with FOB scope.

Fig. 4.11 An ETT extender has been inserted into the LMA to connect to the proximal portion of the endotracheal tube

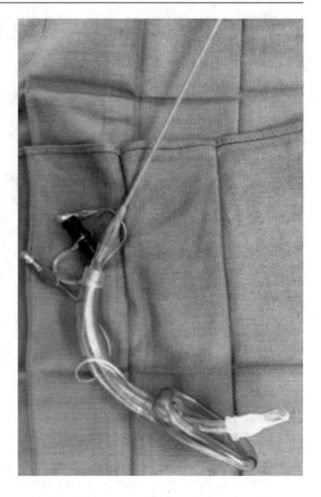

Method #5: Intubating While Ventilating Through an LMA, Using an Aintree Catheter

Equipment
- Intubating LMA
  - Cook LMA: works the best; wide tube to accommodate ETT and FOB scope; short tube length so when scope exists the bowl of LMA, superior enough to see the vocal cords versus so deep that exit directly into the esophagus.
  - LMA Unique: wide tube, longer tube than Cook LMA, less curved; may need to cut the LMA tube to shorten it or use a longer ETT such as a nasal RAE or MLT (microlaryngoscopy tube).
- 5.0 mm FOB scope (large sized)

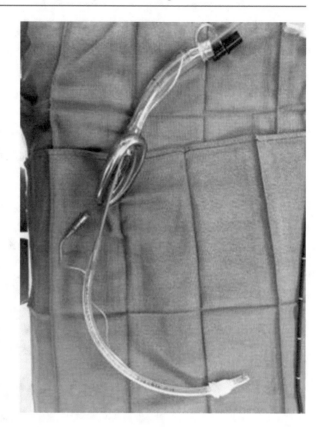

Fig. 4.12 The ETT extender has been used to advance the ETT through the LMA

- 7.0 ETT
  - LMA Unique size 5 will fit a 7.0 ETT
  - LMA Unique size 4 will fit a 6.0 ETT
- Aintree catheter
- Lubricant
- Antifog solution
- Face mask
- Elbow adaptor compatible with FOB scope

Steps
1. Set up FOB scope and tower. Lubricate all equipment and ensure everything slides smoothly over one another.
2. Remove 15 mm adaptor from ETT and tape to ventilator.
3. Set aside the FOB scope and ETT for now.
4. Position patient for intubation.
5. Standard pre-oxygenation with face mask already connected to bronchoscopy elbow adaptor.

Fig. 4.13 The LMA has been removed completely proximally from the ETT extender/ETT setup

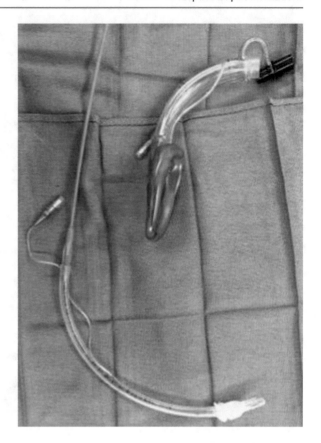

6. Standard IV induction including paralytic. Do not want patient to cough and buck while using the FOB scope.
7. Insert LMA and connect to ventilator circuit and bronchoscopy elbow adaptor (Fig. 4.20).
8. Ensure adequate bag mask ventilation using $ETCO_2$ capnogram.
9. Switch to ventilator at programmed settings and ensure continued appropriate ventilation using $ETCO_2$ capnogram. Keep peak inspiratory pressures as low as possible to avoid filling stomach with gas.
10. Take the FOB scope that has been preloaded with the Aintree catheter.
11. Carefully advance the FOB scope into the elbow adaptor, through the LMA (Fig. 4.21).
12. Advance the FOB scope past the tongue, identify the vocal cords, advance past the cords, and locate the carina.
13. Slide the Aintree catheter over the FOB scope and into the trachea at enough depth that the Aintree will not be easily dislodged.

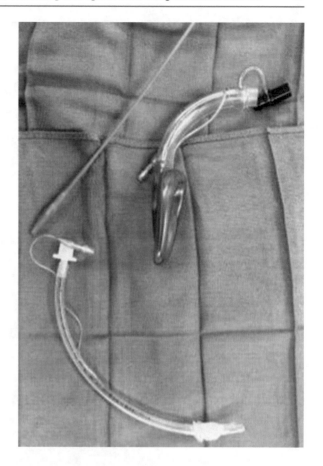

Fig. 4.14 The ETT extender has been disconnected from the ETT and the 15 mm adaptor reattached to the proximal portion of the ETT

14. Pull the FOB scope completely out of the LMA and bronchoscopy elbow adaptor. Be careful not to remove the Aintree.
15. Remove the LMA over the Aintree catheter, being careful to leave the Aintree catheter in the trachea.
16. Slide the ETT over the Aintree and into the trachea. Note the depth of the ETT.
17. Remove the Aintree catheter through the ETT, being careful to leave the ETT in the trachea.
18. Connect ETT to the ventilator circuit and resume ventilation. Verify appropriate $ETCO_2$ capnogram.
19. Reconfirm position of ETT using FOB scope.

Fig. 4.15 If an ETT
extender is not available, a
6.0 ETT with the 15 mm
adaptor removed can be
used instead to advance the
larger ETT
through the LMA

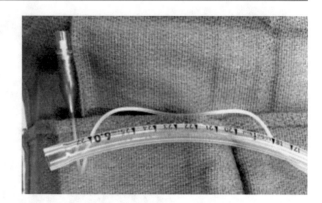

Fig. 4.16 Demonstration
of the 6.0 ETT with the
15 mm adaptor removed,
now attached to the
proximal portion of the 7.0
ETT in the LMA

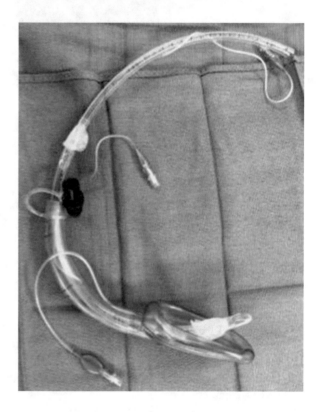

Fig. 4.17 The 6.0 ETT is
used to advance the 7.0
ETT through the LMA

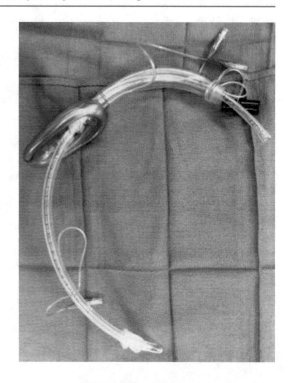

Fig. 4.18 The LMA has
been removed completely
from the 6.0 ETT/7.0 ETT
assembly

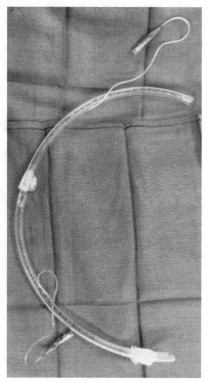

Fig. 4.19 The 6.0 cuffed
ETT used as an ETT
extended detached from
the 7.0 cuffed
ETT and LMA

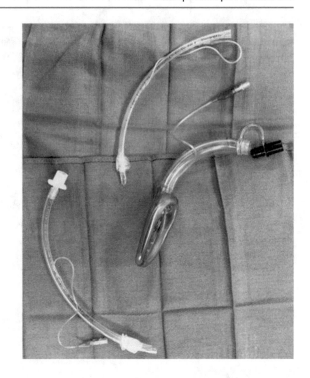

Fig. 4.20 Aintree catheter
preloaded onto the
fiberoptic bronchoscope
(right). Cook LMA
attached to bronchoscopy
elbow adaptor

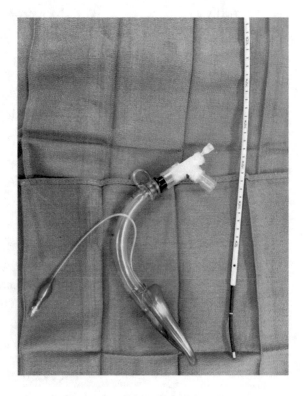

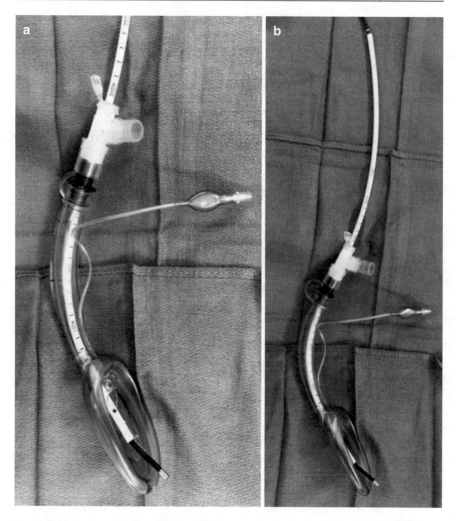

Fig. 4.21 (**a/b**) Aintree catheter loaded over the fiberoptic bronchoscope. Aintree-FOB scope unit passed through an LMA

Awake Fiberoptic Intubation

5

Goals for Awake Fiberoptic Intubation
1. Psychological buy-in
2. Antisialogogue
3. Topicalization
4. Nerve blocks
5. Sedation

Indications for Awake Intubation

- Awake intubation is less desirable than asleep due to patient comfort. However, If you are thinking a patient needs an awake intubation, you should be on alert. Do *not* hesitate to do an awake intubation if it is indicated, as it can save your patient from a lost airway and death or an emergency surgical airway:
- History of difficult intubation
- Suspected difficult intubation due to the following:
  - Trauma to airway, head, and neck
  - Deep neck infections
  - Tumors of larynx or pharynx
  - History of radiation to airway → "woody," stiff neck, poor neck range of motion, poor soft tissue compliance
  - Severe ankylosing spondylitis, arthritis
  - Acromegaly
  - Congenital airway abnormality
  - Inability to access cricothyroid membrane in case emergency surgical airway is required
  - Morbid obesity, obstructive sleep apnea
- High risk for aspiration of gastric contents
- Need for neurological exam immediately following intubation

© The Author(s), under exclusive license to Springer Nature Switzerland AG 2021
C. Sampankanpanich Soria et al., *Anesthesiology Resident Manual of Procedures*,
https://doi.org/10.1007/978-3-030-65732-1_5

Relative Contraindications to Awake Intubation

- Patient refusal
  - Psychiatric illness
  - Acute intoxication with ETOH (alcohol), substance abuse
  - Communication barrier: language, intellectual disability
- Allergy to local anesthetics

But ENT Said It Was Not Necessary...

- Size matters
  - Every tumor has a doubling time.
  - A "small" mass in clinic 2 months ago may be a relatively large mass at the time of surgery.
  - 1 molar tooth = 1 cm × 1 cm × 1 cm = 1 cm^3.
  - A 2 × 2 × 2 cm mass sounds small but = 8 cm^3 = 8 molar teeth in size!
  - Clinical signs that airway mass has grown
      Increased difficulty swallowing
      Increased difficulty breathing, especially when lying down
      Vocal changes
- Context matters
  - ENT surgeons perform flexible indirect laryngoscopies in clinic weeks prior to surgery.
  - A clinic patient is awake, spontaneously ventilating, non-sedated, and non-paralyzed.
  - In the OR under general anesthesia, the patient is asleep, apneic, and paralyzed → loss of pharyngeal tone → cannot mask ventilate + cannot see the vocal cords → loss of airway.
- Airway is a game of millimeters. It is all small changes to get the golden view.

(I) Psychological Buy-In

1. Build trust with the patient.
2. Counsel them about the sequence of events.
3. Emphasize to them that this is uncomfortable, but we will provide IV sedation and numb up the airway as much as possible.
4. Reiterate that this is done for their safety due to anticipated difficult airway.

(II) Antisialogogue

- Purpose: decrease secretions, improve view, and increase adherence of topical local anesthetics.

- Standard medication is glycopyrrolate. Administer glycopyrrolate at least 10–15 min prior to intubation. This can be given in preoperatively before bringing patient back to OR.
- Standard dose is 0.2 mg IV.
- Increase dose to 0.4 mg IV if copious secretions.
- Consider holding or decreasing the dose to 0.1 mg IV if there is underlying cardiac pathology that would be exacerbated by tachycardia (e.g., STEMI, AFib, mitral stenosis).

(III) Topicalization

- Variety of methods by institutional availability and personal preference.
- Can be used solo or in combination.
- Caution with local anesthetic systemic toxicity.
  - Maximum dose of lidocaine w/o epi = 5 mg/kg (Fig. 5.1)
  - Example: 70 kg pt → 5 mg/kg × 70 kg = 350 mg → 350 mg/40 mg/ml (4% lidocaine) = 8.75 cc

Fig. 5.1 Preservative-free lidocaine as a liquid solution

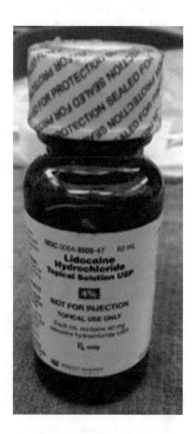

Technique #1: Nebulizer

- Equipment: nebulizer device with spray, handle, bottle to hold lidocaine solution, and tubing to connect to an auxiliary oxygen port (Fig. 5.3).
- Fill up the bottle with preservative-free, 4% lidocaine solution (Fig. 5.1).
- Turn up flow of oxygen to 10 L/min.
- Insert the nebulizer deep into the patient's oropharynx.
- Ask the patient to huff and puff like a dog.
- Spray a little bit of lidocaine solution.
- Then ask the patient to gargle as much solution as possible, then spit it out and suction.
- Press the tip of the nebulizer further and further to the back of the oropharynx and downward, to check if the patient still has a gag reflex.
- Repeat: spray/huff and puff/gargle/spit

Technique #2: Popsicle Stick

- Equipment: 5% Lidocaine ointment on popsicle stick, wrapped with gauze (Figs. 5.2, 5.4 and 5.5)
- Ask patient to suck on the popsicle stick, gargle, swish, spit, and repeat.

Technique #3: Viscous Spray

- Equipment: 2 × 10 cc syringes, 1 stopcock, 1 extension tubing (a PIV pigtail), preservative-free 4% lidocaine, 5% lidocaine jelly or ointment (Fig. 5.5).
- Mix the lidocaine solution and jelly together.
- Aim the pigtail tubing far back into the oropharynx and squirt a small amount. Ask the patient to gargle and swallow/spit it out. Repeat until well-topicalized and able to reach deep/far back into the oropharynx.

(IV) Nerve Blocks

- Not done as commonly anymore
- Contraindications: anticoagulation status

Fig. 5.2 Lidocaine as an ointment

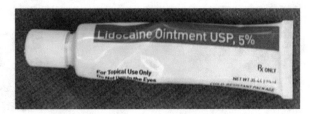

Fig. 5.3 EZ-spray nebulizer device to convert liquid to aerosolized form

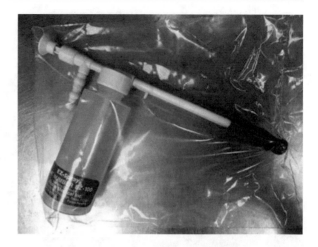

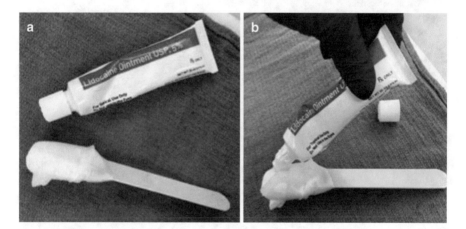

Fig. 5.4 (a/b) Lidocaine ointment on a tongue depressor stick wrapped with gauze

- Glossopharyngeal nerve
- Superior laryngeal nerve
- Transtracheal = Translaryngeal
- Sensory Innervation of the pharynx:
    - Nasopharynx = Trigeminal nerve
    - Oropharynx = Glossopharyngeal nerve
    - Laryngopharynx
        Epiglottis to top of vocal cords = Internal branch of superior laryngeal nerve
        Below vocal cords = Recurrent laryngeal nerve

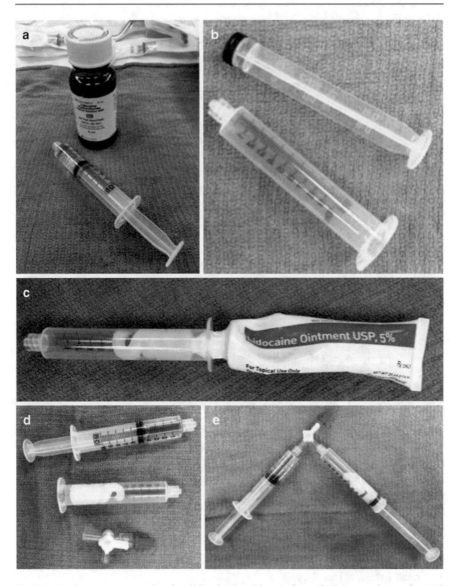

Fig. 5.5 (a) Draw up preservative-free lidocaine in a 10 cc syringe. (b) Remove plunger from 10 cc syringe. (c) Squirt lidocaine ointment into the 10 cc syringe without the plunger. (d) Photo of separate plunger containing lidocaine ointment and syringe with lidocaine liquid. (e) Connect the 10 cc syringe of lidocaine liquid and the 10 cc syringe of lidocaine ointment to a stopcock. (f) Squirt both back and forth with two hands until an even mixture is formed. (g) Connect extension IV tubing (example from a peripheral IV pigtail). Label clearly NOT FOR IV USE

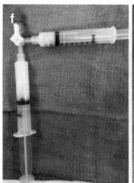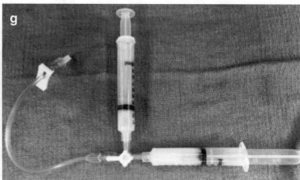

Fig. 5.5 (continued)

Table 5.1 Comparison of pros and cons of common intravenous sedative medications

Drug	Pros	Cons
Midazolam	Bolus 1–2 mg at a time Anxiolysis Short duration of action Fast onset of action Reversible w/Flumazenil	Disinhibition → uncooperative patient Respiratory depression especially when combined with narcotics No analgesia Muscle relaxation → collapsing soft tissues
Fentanyl	Bolus 25–50 mcg at a time Analgesia Reversible w/Naloxone	Respiratory depression especially when combined with benzodiazepines
Dexmedetomidine	Bolus 2–5 mcg at a time or infusion (start low 0.1–0.2 mcg/kg/h) Anxiolysis Unlikely to cause respiratory depression Mild analgesia	Hypotension, bradycardia if administered over <10 min Slow onset of action (10 min) Long duration of action (60–90 min)
Remifentanil	Easily titratable Rapid onset of action Short duration of action Metabolism independent on liver or renal function Bolus 0.25–0.5 mcg/kg at a time and/or infusion 0.1–0.2 mcg/kg/min	Potential for respiratory depression especially when combined with benzodiazepines or longer-acting narcotics

(V) Sedation

- Ideal patient: calm, relaxed, not moving.
- Suboptimal patient: moving, coughing, and grabbing at the provider or FOB scope.
- Choice of IV sedation varies by provider preference (Table 5.1).

Intubation Technique

Equipment
- Fiberoptic tower
- Appropriate-sized fiberoptic scope (usually 5.0 large scope)
- Appropriate-sized ETT (usually 7.0 ETT)
- Antisialogogue (normally glycopyrrolate)
- Induction agents of choice (usually propofol and rocuronium or succinylcholine)
- Elbow adaptor compatible with bronchoscope
- Intubating oral airway (routinely pink 10 cm for men, yellow 9 cm for women; occasionally white Ovassapian)
- Gauze to manually retract patient's tongue
- Lubricant
- Antifog solution
- Back-up airway equipment
  - Various sized blades
  - Various sized ETTs
  - Cook LMA
  - Cricothyrotomy kit
- Suction
- Monitors
- Nasal cannula connected to auxiliary O_2 port
- Preservative-free 4% lidocaine on a 10 cc slip-tip syringe

Recommended method: if the airway has been well anesthetized, the patient will tolerate an intubating oral airway. This makes it easier for the provider and only necessitates one anesthesia provider.

Steps
1. Recommended setting: operating room, with extra OR RN, anesthesia tech, and/or second anesthesia provider. Depending on the case, may want ENT or trauma surgery scrubbed, prepped, and draped for emergency tracheostomy if awake intubation fails.
2. Set up FOB scope and tower. Lubricate all equipment and ensure everything slides smoothly over one another.
3. Remove the 15 mm adaptor from the endotracheal tube and place this in a secure location. (Usually taped to the ventilator or FOB tower.)
4. Pre-load the endotracheal tube onto the FOB scope. Secure to the scope handle using a strip of tape or a rubber band.
5. Obtain psychological buy-in.
6. Administer antisialogogue at least 10–15 min prior to topicalization.
7. Proceed with airway anesthetization: topicalization or nerve blocks.
8. Once airway is well anesthetized, proceed with intubation.
9. Start additional IV sedation if desired.

10. Connect propofol and rocuronium or succinylcholine syringes in line. As soon as ETT is in, can induce patient and minimize patient coughing, bucking, and distress.
11. Where to stand
    (a) Personal preference
    (b) Provider stands facing patient/head of bed
        (i) Improves face-to-face communication
        (ii) Disorienting because image is reversed from traditional view
        (iii) How to make scope orientation easier: hold the scope the same way ENT surgeons do. Continue to hold the scope in standard format, such that turning clockwise turns to *provider's* right; pushing lever down will flex scope anterior to *provider*. Right of screen is patient's left, but this becomes irrelevant. The target is still the trachea.
    (c) Provider stands at head of bed, facing the feet
        (i) Standard position, traditional views of airway
12. Position the patient for intubation: flat chest, room for head extension, and tragus in line with sternum. Recommend elevate head of bed for patient comfort.
13. Place nasal cannula over the patient to provide supplemental oxygen while the patient is spontaneously ventilating.
14. Advance fiberoptic scope into oropharynx and identify vocal cords.
15. With the scope just proximal to the vocal cords, squirt lidocaine down the scope to spray the cords and minimize patient coughing.
16. Advance the scope past the vocal cords and into trachea. Confirm trachea by visualization of cartilaginous rings (vs. esophagus: longitudinal striations).
17. At this point, the patient will begin coughing and bucking more aggressively. Induce the patient with propofol and muscle relaxant, secure the ETT, verify ETT positioning, and proceed with case.

Nasotracheal Intubation

6

Nasal Intubation by Direct Laryngoscopy

Equipment (Fig. 6.1)
1. 7.0 nasal RAE
2. MAC3
3. Magill forceps
4. Afrin (oxymetazoline) spray
5. Warm bottle of saline
6. Surgical lubricant/jelly or lidocaine ointment
7. Nasal trumpets of various sizes (26, 28, 30, 32, 34 Fr), lubricated with surgilube or lidocaine ointment

Fig. 6.1 Equipment for nasal intubations: lubricated nasal trumpets of increasing sizes, lidocaine ointment, warmed and lubricated nasal RAE, Afrin nasal spray, and Magill forceps

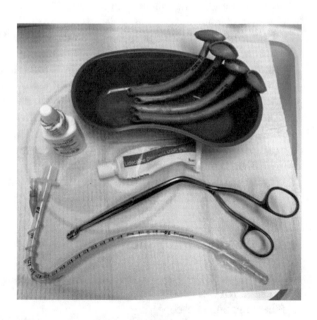

Instructions
1. Place the nasal RAE in warm saline water, distal end first, to soften the tube.
2. Spray Afrin into patient's nose while awake to allow time for onset of action. Ask patient to confirm which nare is more widely patent.
3. Position patient optimally for intubation (flat chest, tragus in line with sternum, room for head extension).
4. Pre-oxygenate.
5. Administer induction agents.
6. One after the other, insert nasal trumpets in increasing size down one nare.
   (a) Ideally use the left nare, so the bevel of the nasal trumpet faces laterally away from the nasal turbinates, decreasing the risk of trauma.
   (b) If the nasal trumpet does not pass easily through the left nare, then use the right nare.
7. Remove the nasal RAE from the warm saline. Coat with surgilube or lidocaine ointment.
8. Carefully insert the nasal RAE empirically to a depth of 18 cm at the nare.
   (a) 15 cm from nares to epiglottis
   (b) 3 cm from epiglottis to vocal cords
   (c) =18 cm from nares to vocal cords
9. Perform direct laryngoscopy with left hand.
10. After scissoring and obtaining view, pick up Magill forceps with right hand, keep forceps closed until they are touching the ETT. When open, they can easily damage mucosa (e.g., uvula, tonsils) or ETT cuff from incidental contact.
11. Identify vocal cords, and gently grasp the tip of the ETT with the Magill forceps.
    (a) Caution: Do not grab the cuff, as you may tear the cuff.
    (b) Do not grab the tonsils with the Magill forceps, as this may cause trauma and bleeding.
12. Advance the ETT through the vocal cords with the Magill forceps, cuff to go 1–2 cm past the cords.
13. Ensure the ETT seats well. If the patient is too tall and the nasal RAE is too short, the ETT can easily become dislodged.
14. Attach straight connector and ETT extension to the nasal RAE.
15. Discuss ETT securement with the surgeons. Oftentimes, ENT surgeons have their own preferred technique for securing the ETT.
    (a) Example: small piece of foam placed between the ETT and the patient's nose to minimize trauma to the nose.
    (b) Strip of foam tape placed underneath the patient's head and wrapped around the ETT/circuit extension.

Nasal Fiberoptic Intubation

Equipment
1. 7.0 nasal RAE
2. Fiberoptic bronchoscope

3. Afrin (oxymetazoline) spray
4. Warm bottle of saline
5. Surgical lubricant/jelly or lidocaine ointment
6. Nasal trumpets of various sizes (26, 28, 30, 32, 34 Fr) lubricated with surgilube or lidocaine ointment

Instructions

1. Prepare the FOB scope. Lubricate all equipment.
2. Place the nasal RAE in warm saline water, distal end first, to soften the tube.
3. Spray Afrin into patient's nose while awake to allow time for onset of action, ask patient to confirm which nare is more widely patent.
4. Position patient optimally for intubation (flat chest, tragus in line with sternum, room for head extension).
5. Pre-oxygenate.
6. Administer induction agents.
7. One after the other, insert nasal trumpets in increasing size down one nare.
   (a) Ideally use the left nare, so the bevel of the nasal trumpet faces laterally away from the nasal turbinates, decreasing the risk of trauma.
   (b) If the nasal trumpet does not pass easily through the left nare, then use the right nare.
8. Remove the nasal RAE from the warm saline. Coat with surgilube or lidocaine ointment.
9. Carefully insert the nasal RAE empirically to a depth of 18 cm at the nare (Fig. 6.2)/(Fig. 6.3).

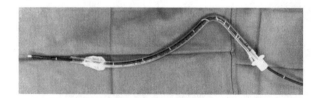

Fig. 6.2 Fiberoptic bronchoscope inserted through a nasal endotracheal tube

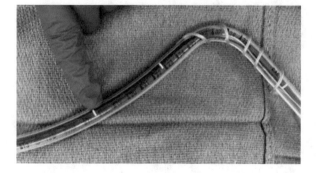

Fig. 6.3 Marker indicating 18 cm depth of nasal endotracheal tube, with fiberoptic bronchoscope inserted through the ETT

10. Insert the FOB scope through the nasal RAE. Scope should exit just outside the vocal cords.
    (a) If the ETT is too deep, the scope will likely enter into the esophagus.
    (b) If the ETT is too high up, the scope will have a couple centimeters to traverse to reach the vocal cords.
11. Guide FOB scope through the vocal cords, down the trachea, to reach carina.
12. Slide the ETT over the scope.
13. As you remove the FOB scope, ensure you visualize trachea and then ETT.
14. Secure ETT.

Codes/Out of or Emergency Airway Management

7

Assess the Patient

(1) Vital Signs
- Is the patient actively desaturating?
  - Yes → secure airway as soon as possible
  - No → more time to assess situation
- Is the patient hemodynamically stable?
  - Hypotensive, tachycardic?
- Is the patient actively coding?
  - Yes: Cardiac arrest, pulmonary arrest → secure airway as soon as possible
  - No: Pre-emptive/prophylactic intubation → time to assess situation

(2) Airway
- Is the airway patent?
  - Is the patient already intubated? – confirm ETT placement with capnography AND breath sounds (Mainstem intubation? Pneumothorax?), troubleshoot existing ETT
  - Trauma, hematoma, angioedema (lips, tongue, facial swelling)
  - Evidence of obstruction – audible stridor, obese, pregnant, large thick neck
  - Tracheostomy – Why? How long? Is it useable? Is the native airway accessible through the oropharynx – i.e., is direct laryngoscopy feasible?

(3) Breathing
- Is the patient breathing? – chest rise, fogging of face mask, presence of $ETCO_2$, audible breath sounds, speech
- Auscultation – inspiratory stridor, expiratory wheezing, absence of breath sounds on one side (pneumothorax, hemothorax, pleural effusion), crackles (pulmonary edema, interstitial lung disease)

(4) Circulation
- Is there a pulse?
- Is the patient hemodynamically stable?

© The Author(s), under exclusive license to Springer Nature Switzerland AG 2021
C. Sampankanpanich Soria et al., *Anesthesiology Resident Manual of Procedures*,
https://doi.org/10.1007/978-3-030-65732-1_7

MOMSAID for Out of OR Situations

Bring all anticipated necessary airway equipment to the head of the bed. Never assume that a non-anesthesia provider will know what equipment to hand you.

(1) Machine
   - Mapleson D circuit
     - Advantages
       Adjust pop-off valve to deliver PEEP/CPAP
       Compliance of bag
       - Bag not filling: leak vs. tight seal w/face mask
       - Stiff compliance: obstructive/restrictive ventilatory defect
       Optimal to maximize gas flow and minimize rebreathing in spontaneously and manually ventilated patients
     - Disadvantages
       Only used by anesthesia providers
       Tricky to adjust pop-off valve
       Bag won't inflate unless tight seal w/face mask
       Requires fresh gas flow, NOT self-inflating
       Not found throughout the hospital; only anesthesiologists carry them
   - Ambu-Bag
     - Advantages
       Self-inflating
       Easy to use
       Hangs in bag w/face mask on O_2 tree in every hospital room, underneath gurneys w/O_2 tank
     - Disadvantages
       No tactile feedback on lung compliance
       No tactile feedback on adequate mask seal
(2) Oxygen
   - Out of OR, any hospital bed: wall O_2, central supply
   - Out of OR, out of hospital bed (hallway, waiting room, pharmacy): portable O_2 tank
   - Ideally pre-oxygenate × 3–5 min; de-nitrogenate, fill up Functional Residual Capacity (FRC) w/O_2; desaturate less quickly
   - How long will your tank last? 1 full tank = 2000 psi = 660 L (at 10 L/min, full tank will last about 1 h)
(3) Monitor
   - Transport monitor or monitor in room
   - Pulse oximeter
     - Ensure pulse oximeter has good waveform for accurate reading
     - At SpO_2 <80%, highly inaccurate reading b/c lack of calibration
     - Manually turn on pulse oximeter sound on monitor: pitch matches SpO_2 value
   - Cycle BP cuff q1min or use arterial line if available

- EKG
  - Ideally 5-lead EKG; 3-lead acceptable
  - If no EKG available, use poor man's pulse from pulse oximeter
- ETCO$_2$
  - Capnometer: color change (purple to gold) with pH change (decreased pH w/CO$_2$)
    - Caution: will not see color change if not perfusing adequately (e.g., inadequate chest compressions)
  - Quantitative ETCO$_2$ measurement: ideal, not always available out of OR
(4) Suction
  - Out of OR, any hospital bed: wall suction; always have available before intubating!
  - Anticipate the unexpected: bloody airways, emesis, mucus/secretions – obstruct view.
  - Out of OR, out of hospital bed (e.g., pharmacy, courtyard, lobby): no suction available unless ED brings their cart with portable suction.
(5) Airway
  - Masking a patient
    - Don't usually mask if Rapid Sequence Induction (RSI) B/c full-stomach, aspiration risk (out of OR, everyone is presumed full-stomach). HOWEVER, if patient is desaturating and you have not been able to intubate, then you absolutely should mask ventilate or place LMA if necessary. If you are not able to preoxygenate a patient (e.g., uncooperative patient in trauma bay), then do not hesitate to mask ventilate while cricoid pressure is applied until patient is intubated.
    - When to mask: patient not spontaneously ventilating; in between intubation attempts; desaturating as above.
    - Techniques to improve mask ventilation
      - Chin lift
      - Jaw thrust
      - Shoulder roll
      - Oral airway
      - Nasal trumpet
      - One-handed vs. two-handed technique
    - Sources of leaks
      - Lack of tight seal – provider technique
      - Mask doesn't conform to face – one size doesn't fit all
      - Beards and moustaches – shave if needed; use tegaderms to create tight seal w/face mask
      - OG (orogastric) or NG (nasogastric) tubes – removal of pre-intubation is controversial; suction them before intubation to minimize aspiration risk
  - Airway adjuncts
    - Oral airway, tongue blade

- – Nasal trumpet, surgical jelly – caution w/head trauma, potential basilar skull fractures, already have bloody nasopharynx/orbital fracture/nasal fracture
- Deciding the method of intubation
  - – Direct laryngoscopy
    Most adult patients: MAC 3 or 4, 7.0 ETT (8.0 ETT if patients need bronchoscopic clearance of secretions (e.g., inhalation injury, severe pneumonia))
  - – Glidescope
    Unstable C-spine; known/anticipated difficult airway; anterior view on DL/unable to pass Bougie
    Not always readily available out of OR or ICU
  - – Fiberoptic intubation
    Awake vs. asleep – Can you mask the patient? Risk of aspiration – need to be awake to maintain protective reflexes?
    Nasal vs. oral
  - – Can't intubate, can't ventilate
    LMA
    - • Proper placement can be tricky
    - • Temporizing measure until secure airway
    - • Aspiration risk
    - • Fiberoptic intubation through Cook LMA easier – stiff, wide lumen but can intubate through any LMA
    Surgical airway – cricothyrotomy
    12 or 14 G needle, jet ventilate (available in OR)
    Wake patient up – on average, induction agents wear off in ~10 min; succinylcholine wears off in ~10 min; rocuronium – sugammadex reversal in several minutes (institutional availability) but you'll likely still be waiting for hypnotics to wear off
- Bougie in back pocket in case of grade 3 view
- Optimize patient positioning
  - – Patients often sunken into hospital beds, covered with food trays, blankets, gowns, TV remotes, phones
  - – Shoulder roll
    Rolled blanket
    Pillow folded in half
  - – Bring patient close to head of bed to improve ergonomics
  - – Flatten head of bed vs. slightly elevate – relieve abdominal pressure
  - – Optimal sniffing position
    Flat chest (obese, pregnant, large breasts)
    Tragus in line with sternum
    Room for head extension
  - – Difficult if C-spine precautions

Remove anterior portion of C-collar + surgeon holds cervical in-line stabilization

Keep the entire C-collar on

(6) IV
- Establish functional IV access, bolus line, flushes

(7) Drugs
- Hemodynamically unstable – hypotensive, tachycardic
  - Etomidate: causes less hypotension; risk of myoclonus, nausea/emesis, burning sensation in vein on administration, decreases seizure threshold, even single dose can suppress adrenal function; in septic/adrenally depleted patient, it can cause profound hypotension refractory to resuscitation
  - Note on propofol: causes hypotension from myocardial stunning, systemic vasodilatation – loss of preload and afterload; use out of OR varies by patient and institution
  - Opioids and benzodiazipines: in severe cases of hemodynamic instability where even cautious dosing of etomidate or propofol may precipitate hemodynamic collapse (e.g., massive hemorrhage, acute right ventricular failure), it is possible to solely administer opioids and benzodiazepines as induction agents. Narcotics provide analgesia and blunt the hemodynamic response to intubation. However, they provide limited hypnosis; thus, benzodiazepines are commended for anxiolysis and amnesia.
- Paralytic
  - Succinylcholine: depolarizing neuromuscular blocker (NMB); fastest acting paralytic (30 s); short duration of action <10 min – can perform neurologic exam soon after intubation (e.g., stroke, seizure patient); fasciculations cause muscle soreness; contraindications – demyelinating injury (stroke, spinal cord injury); muscular dystrophy; severe abdominal infections; rhabdomyolysis, crush injuries, prolonged immobilization → severe hyperkalemia → VTach/VFib/cardiac arrest; penetrating eye injury (causes increased intraocular pressure)
  - Rocuronium: non-depolarizing NMB; second fastest acting after succinylcholine (30–60 s); longer duration of action; reversible with sugammadex (institutional availability)

Airway Exchanges

8

Indications

1. Increasing to large-sized ETT
   (a) Prolonged intubation in ICU
   (b) Repeated bronchoscopies
   (c) Bleeding from ETT
   (d) Going prone, protect against kinking (e.g., armored ETT)
2. Exchange for new, clean ETT
   (a) Old ETT clotted off with blood, mucous plugs, secretions
3. Malfunctioning
   (a) Pilot bulb torn off → cuff leak
   (b) Cuff torn
   (c) Kinked ETT
4. Staged extubation
   (a) Plan to extubate patient at end of case, but concerned about possible need for reintubation which could be difficult
   (b) Difficult intubation at start of case
   (c) Edematous airway (e.g., prone surgery with large volume fluid administration)

Settings
1. Operating room
2. ICU
3. Burn center

© The Author(s), under exclusive license to Springer Nature Switzerland AG 2021
C. Sampankanpanich Soria et al., *Anesthesiology Resident Manual of Procedures*,
https://doi.org/10.1007/978-3-030-65732-1_8

Airway Exchange Devices

Method

1. Airway exchange (Table 8.1)
   (a) Position patient for intubation: flat chest, tragus in line with sternum, room for head extension.
   (b) Pre-oxygenate: 100% FiO_2 on current ventilator settings.
   (c) Easiest to perform with second assisting provider.
   (d) Direct laryngoscopy to obtain at least grade 2 view. Must be able to visualize the ETT and AEC sitting in the cords.
   (e) Disconnect old ETT from ventilator circuit.
   (f) Insert AEC through old ETT. Do not advance AEC more than 26 cm at the teeth (15 cm teeth to vocal cords +10–12 cm trachea):
       (i) Right mainstem intubation
       (ii) Airway perforation
       (iii) Rigid small diameter catheter ventilating 1 of 2 lungs
       (iv) No time for egress of air
   (g) Remove old ETT.
   (h) Slide new ETT over the AEC.
   (i) If meet resistance, likely hung up on arytenoids. Rotate counterclockwise with only gentle pressure on ETT.
   (j) Visualize the ETT going through the vocal cords (VCs).
   (k) Remove AEC.
2. Jet Ventilation
   (a) Maximum pressure of 15–18 psi.
   (b) Maximum 0.5 s duration of inspiration to minimize risk of barotrauma.
   (c) With an AEC, one can achieve total volumes of 400 cc.
   (d) Watch chest rise and fall. Ensure enough time to allow for expiration.
   (e) Maintain upper airway patency using bilateral nasal trumpets, oral airway, chin lift, and bilateral jaw thrust. Cannot rely solely on passive expiration through a small conduit. Need air to go out and around the AEC as well.
3. Using the AEC for ventilation:
   (a) Ideally, done in OR with access to jet ventilation.
   (b) AECs come with adaptor to connect AEC to standard Mapleson, Ambu Bag, ventilator circuit (Fig 8.1).

Table 8.1 Comparison of the pros and cons of an airway exchange catheter versus a Bougie

Device	Pros	Cons
Airway exchange catheter (AEC)	Can ventilate using AEC if unable to pass new ETT (temporizing measure)	Expensive
		Not readily available
	Designed for airway exchanges	outside of the OR
Bougie	Cheap	Cannot ventilate using
	Readily available in trauma bay, OR	Bougie

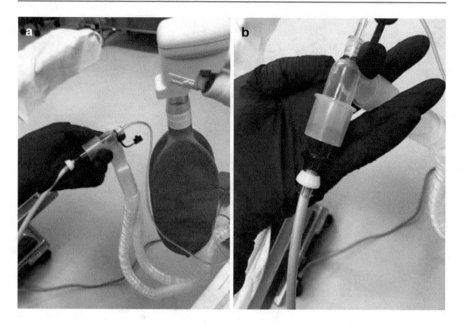

Fig. 8.1 (**a/b**) Demonstration of adaptor used to connect Aintree catheter to a ventilator circuit for ventilation

    (c) Rate-limiting factor is time and space for expiration, as the lumens to the AECs are much smaller than a standard ETT. Bilateral jaw thrust, chin lift, oral airway, and nasal trumpets should be inserted, and the chest should be watched carefully to ensure air is released. Otherwise, the patient will auto-PEEP, leading quickly to severe volutrauma and barotrauma.

4. Maintaining the AEC

    (a) Scenario: worried about extubating a patient completely. Remove the ETT over an AEC. Leave the AEC in the airway as a conduit to facilitate emergency re-intubation.

    (b) Technique:

        (i) Insert AEC through current ETT, maximum depth of 26 cm at teeth.

        (ii) Remove ETT with AEC in place.

        (iii) Graduated removal of AEC a couple centimeter at a time. Continue removal if patient tolerates ventilation on their own.

        (iv) If one chooses to keep AEC in place, topicalize the airway by squirting preservative-free lidocaine down the AEC. This can also be done prior to removing ETT. Most patients will tolerate the AEC well.

    (c) Risks: aspiration. Airway is anesthetized, inhibiting protective airway reflexes. Foreign object is sitting directly between the vocal cords, so they are not closed off completely from aspiration.

Deep Extubations

9

Indications

1. Minimize risk of bronchospasm
2. Minimize coughing and bucking on ETT
   - (a) → Increased intracranial pressure → intracerebral hemorrhage
   - (b) → Increased intraocular pressure → globe (re-)rupture
   - (c) → Increased oral/nasal venous pressure → bleeding after ENT surgery/ESS/etc.
   - (d) → Increased intra-abdominal pressure → suture tear, bowel (re-)herniation
3. Enable gentle, smooth emergence in an anxious patient

Contraindications

1. Difficult intubation
2. Full stomach/high risk of aspiration
   - (a) NPO status
   - (b) Pregnant
   - (c) Morbidly obese
   - (d) Diabetic, gastroparesis
   - (e) Bowel obstruction
3. Blood in the stomach or oropharynx
   - (a) ENT/neurosurgery – operating on the mouth or nose, must be completely "dry" if attempting deep extubation to avoid risk of vocal cord irritation/laryngospasm/aspiration
   - (b) Highly recommend passing OG tube to suction blood from stomach

© The Author(s), under exclusive license to Springer Nature Switzerland AG 2021
C. Sampankanpanich Soria et al., *Anesthesiology Resident Manual of Procedures*,
https://doi.org/10.1007/978-3-030-65732-1_9

Technique

1. Patient must be spontaneously ventilating off the ventilator with appropriate respiratory rate, tidal volume, and $ETCO_2$.
2. Anesthetic: 1 full mean alveolar concentration (MAC) of volatile anesthetic, 100% FiO_2.
3. Place oral airway and/or nasal trumpet prior to extubation. Important to avoid obstruction after extubation as it is very stimulating to airway and increases risk of laryngospasm.
4. Suction the oropharynx very well. Secretions = laryngospasm.
5. Position patient in optimal position prior to extubation.
6. Prepare all emergency airway backup equipment. Must be available within arms' reach, especially if you're by yourself.
   (a) Propofol 20 cc × 1
   (b) Succinylcholine 10 cc × 1
   (c) Oral airway
   (d) Face mask
   (e) Blade and tube for reintubation
7. Verify whether patient is deeply anesthetized
   (a) Methods of stimulation:
       (i) Suction oropharynx deep
       (ii) Jiggle the ETT
       (iii) Bilateral jaw thrust
   (b) No cough or gag reflex
   (c) No change in respiratory pattern (e.g., breath holding) with stimulation
       (i) Sometimes the cough or gag reflex is delayed, and patient only demonstrates a change in ventilatory pattern
8. How to deepen the patient to assist with deep extubation
   (a) 1 full MAC of volatile anesthetic
   (b) Fentanyl
   (c) Dexmedetomidine
   (d) Propofol
   (e) Lidocaine
9. When ready for deep extubation…
10. Extubate on 100% FiO_2, 10 L/min O_2, 1 MAC volatile anesthetic (*note that deep extubation can also be accomplished from a Total Intravenous Anesthetic (TIVA)
11. Suction oropharynx again.
12. Ensure oral airway and/or nasal trumpet in place.
13. Place face mask on patient immediately.
14. Provide chin lift and jaw thrust. Tight seal with face mask.
15. Confirm whether patient is still spontaneously ventilating by checking $ETCO_2$ capnogram.
16. Look for signs of airway obstruction or laryngospasm:

    (a) Audible inspiratory stridor

    (b) Pulling at sternal notch and supraclavicular area

    (c) Paradoxical abdominal movements (abdomen pushes out with inspiration)

    (d) Absence of fogging of face mask

    (e) Absence of ETCO$_2$

17. IF ventilating well, turn off sevoflurane completely. Continue 100% FiO$_2$, 10 L/min O$_2$.

    (a) Option 1: Gradually release chin lift and jaw thrust to see if patient ventilates without manual assistance.

    (b) Option 2: Continue to hold chin lift and jaw thrust until patient has gone through stage 2. Preventing any degree of airway obstruction can help decrease stimulation of the larynx which may cause laryngospasm.

18. IF there is airway obstruction:

    (a) Do NOT leave the OR

    (b) Assistive maneuvers

       (i) Chin lift

       (ii) Jaw thrust

       (iii) Head extension/shoulder roll

    (c) Airway adjuncts

       (i) Nasal trumpet × 2

       (ii) Oral airway

19. IF there is laryngospasm

    (a) Do NOT leave the OR. Consider calling for help.

    (b) All patients

       (i) Tight face mask seal

       (ii) Assistive maneuvers + airway adjuncts

    (c) First line: Positive pressure breaths to manually break the laryngospasm and open vocal cords.

    (d) Second line: Deepen with propofol 20–30 mg or re-paralyze with succinylcholine 10–20 mg.

       (i) The exact dosing of propofol and/or succinylcholine depends on the severity of the laryngospasm.

       (ii) In general, the goal is to deepen the patient fast enough which may require you to mask ventilate them briefly.

       (iii) If deepening the patient with propofol does not open the vocal cords right away, you will need to administer paralytic quickly. Succinylcholine 10–20 mg may suffice, or higher doses at 1–2 mg/kg may be required if the laryngospasm is severe and you are heading toward reintubation.

       (iv) It is important to have propofol and succinylcholine syringes already drawn up and easily accessible in the event of laryngospasm. You need to work quickly to avoid negative pressure pulmonary edema and hypoxia from a patient spontaneously ventilating against closed vocal cords.

    (e) Third line: reintubate

20. Stage 2 and emergence
    (a) Emerge in OR
        (i) Safest location
        (ii) If there are any concerns with airway during or after deep extubation, allow patient to awaken in OR.
    (b) Transporting to PACU (only if smooth extubation/good airway in OR)
        (i) Bring a mapleson and face mask so that in case of emergency, you can take over positive pressure ventilation.
        (ii) Keep a stick of propofol and a stick of succinylcholine in your pocket.
        (iii) When in doubt, return to the OR.
    (c) Emerge in PACU
        (i) Strongly advised not to leave a patient in PACU until they have emerged from stage 2.
        (ii) Remain with patient and continue to observe carefully for signs of airway obstruction.

Aspiration on Induction

10

Risk Factors

1. Nil per os (NPO) status
2. Delayed gastric emptying:
   (a) Pregnant
   (b) Poorly controlled diabetes mellitus
   (c) Pain, narcotic use
3. High intra-abdominal pressure
   (a) Bowel obstruction
   (b) Obese
   (c) Pregnant
   (d) Ascites

Preventive Measures

1. Rapid sequence induction = no mask ventilation
2. Cricoid pressure: controversial
   - There is insufficient evidence to advocate or abandon cricoid pressure for prevention of passive regurgitation in at-risk patients.
   - Potential benefits include minimizing gastric distention and lessening risk of aspiration.
   - Potential risks include impaired gas exchange and ventilation.
   - It remains standard of care to provide cricoid pressure.
   - Properly timed and properly applied, it may provide benefit and is unlikely to cause any significant harm.
   - Cricoid pressure should be released if there is any difficulty in either intubating or ventilating the patient.

© The Author(s), under exclusive license to Springer Nature Switzerland AG 2021
C. Sampankanpanich Soria et al., *Anesthesiology Resident Manual of Procedures*,
https://doi.org/10.1007/978-3-030-65732-1_10

3. Caution with benzodiazepines and narcotics prior to induction
   - Classically, it was recommended to avoid opioids and benzodiazepines because of theoretical respiratory depression or nausea/vomiting.
   - In the setting of pain and anxiety, though, prudent use of these agents has been safely accomplished.

What if Patient Vomits Right Before Induction?

1. Empties stomach while patient is still awake and has intact protective airway reflexes.
2. Danger: there may still be more potential emesis upon induction.
3. Strongly consider prophylactically placing a nasogastric tube and suctioning the stomach prior to induction.
   (a) Example scenarios:
      (i) Gastrointestinal pathology like small bowel obstruction
      (ii) Delayed gastric emptying: poorly controlled diabetes, significant pain and narcotic use
   (b) Cons:
      (i) Patient discomfort
      (ii) Time delay in emergency case
      (iii) Controversial whether to remove the NG tube after suctioning and prior to induction. Theoretically stomach has already been emptied now. Presence of NG tube prevents complete closure of the upper and lower esophageal sphincters
   (c) Pros:
      (i) Empties stomach
      (ii) Can be left in place for continued suctioning postoperatively (e.g., remain intubated in ICU)

What if Patients Vomits/Aspirates upon/After Induction?

1. If patient is already asleep, suction oropharynx very well.
2. Quickly obtain secure airway as fast as possible: ideally intubate on first attempt without mask ventilating and then suction through ETT in case gastric contents might be removed.
3. Head of bed down to prevent gastric contents from moving by gravity from oropharynx into the airway.
4. Place orogastric tube after intubation and suction out the stomach.
5. 100% FiO_2, wean as tolerated.
6. High PEEP ~8 cm H_2O.
7. Check arterial blood gas.

8. Fiberoptic bronchoscopy in OR: bronchoalveolar lavage with saline.
9. Chest X-ray postoperative, may be useful especially if large particles of food have been aspirated and obstruction of large airways is apparent.
10. Consider keeping patient intubated due to concerns for development of aspiration pneumonia or pneumonitis a few days later.

Intubating Without Muscle Relaxant

11

Indications

- Necessity for motor nerve monitoring during procedure
- Short, quick procedure where:
  - (1) Want to avoid non-depolarizing neuromuscular blockade because will not have adequate return of twitches for reversal before the surgery is done.
    AND
  - (2) Succinylcholine is contraindicated.
- Note that children are often intubated without muscle relaxant after a mask induction where a deep plane of anesthesia has been reached.

Technique

Alfentanil OR remifentanil + propofol + sevoflurane

- Alfentanil 30–100 mcg/kg (Use LBW for obese patients; decrease dose in elderly)
  - Potent
  - Short duration of action: 10–20 min depending upon dose
- Remifentanil 1.5–4 mcg/kg
  - Potent
  - Short duration of action: 3–5 min
- Note on synthetic opioids
  - Profound analgesia of airway, decreases reactivity of glottis to intubation
  - All carry risk of muscle rigidity/laryngospasm/laryngeal closure, especially with rapid high-dose infusion. "Reversed" w/ naloxone or paralytic
- Use of routine hypnotics

© The Author(s), under exclusive license to Springer Nature Switzerland AG 2021
C. Sampankanpanich Soria et al., *Anesthesiology Resident Manual of Procedures*,
https://doi.org/10.1007/978-3-030-65732-1_11

- Mask ventilation with sevoflurane
  - Muscle relaxant properties of volatile anesthetics
  - With children, sevoflurane alone is generally enough to allow for intubation. With larger children and adults, achieving a deep plane of anesthesia is delayed and readiness for intubation after mask induction can be augmented with opioid and/or propofol administration

Confirming Patient Is Anesthetized and Deep Enough for Intubation

1. Eyelid/lash reflex
2. Mandible feels loose, ventilation often feels "easier" as well
3. No response when laryngoscope blade inserted

Jet Ventilation for ENT Surgery

12

Indications

- Discuss with ENT surgeon
- Shared airway
- No secure airway, no ETT, no LMA
- Surgeon operating on the airway

Induction

- Surgeons usually position patient. No typical sniffing position for intubation. Often hyperextended, caution if any spinal stenosis, atlantoaxial instability, or other c-spine abnormalities.
- Pre-oxygenate patient.
- Place nasal cannula to provide supplemental, passive oxygenation (do not do this if laser surgery due to fire risk).
- Induce with propofol and vecuronium – dosed to TOF 1. (Note that in patients who can tolerate high doses of propofol and opioids, paralysis may not be needed.)
- Mask ventilate until gradually TOF decreases from 4 to 1.
- Connect TIVA: propofol gtt and remifentanil gtt. No inhaled anesthetics.
- When ready, hand over airway to surgeons.

Maintenance

- Surgeons will perform rigid bronchoscopy with Parsons scope.
- Jet ventilation connects to a side port on the scope. For suspended laryngoscopy, a Hunsaker jet ventilation endotracheal tube can be placed (Figs. 12.1 and 12.2).

© The Author(s), under exclusive license to Springer Nature Switzerland AG 2021
C. Sampankanpanich Soria et al., *Anesthesiology Resident Manual of Procedures*,
https://doi.org/10.1007/978-3-030-65732-1_12

Fig. 12.1 Handle and
adaptor for jet ventilator,
located on the back of the
ventilator in the
operating room

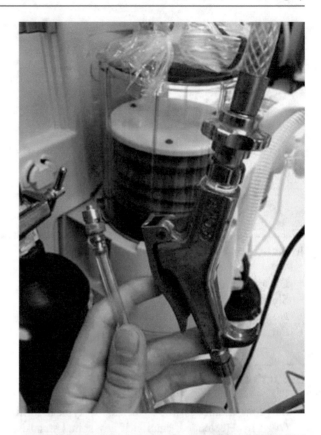

Fig. 12.2 Pressure gauge
for jet ventilator. Adjust
pressure using the dial on
the side. Typical pressures
are 25–35 psi after the jet
ventilator is connected to
the adaptor to be used for
ventilation

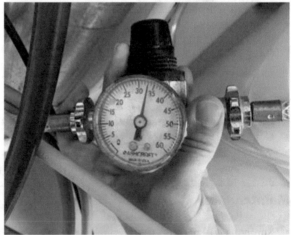

- Clarify with surgeons when it is ok to ventilate and when to hold ventilation.
- Jet ventilation not only delivers 100% FiO_2 but also entrains air. Not able to titrate the FiO_2.
- Hold jet ventilation when cautery or laser to decrease fire risk.
- Technique for jet ventilation
  - Dial pressure gauge to 15–30 psi (comes off main supply at 50 psi)
  - Frequency: 0.5 s inspiration, and enough time for expiration, watch chest rise and fall
  - Standard: 1-2-3-4, ventilate on 1, pause and expiration on 2-3-4
- Frequently check twitches to keep weak but reversible state, TOF 1
  - Do not want patient to cough/gag from operating on vocal cords. Tight surgical space. No room for error.
  - Reversible state: when surgeons are done, that's it. There's nothing to close.
- Caution: expect SpO_2 will drop.
- Avoid jet ventilation for extended periods of time, generally <30 min.
- Large gradient between $ETCO_2$ and $PaCO_2$
- Active oxygenation, passive ventilation

Intubating with a Bougie

13

Why Would I Need a Bougie?

1. Poor laryngeal view with direct laryngoscopy and video laryngoscope, or FOB scope not available – e.g., broken, bad outlet, institutional availability, out of OR, out of ICU.
2. Bougie is very portable and thus can be available everywhere – OR, code bag, ICU, Emergency Room.

When to Use a Bougie

1. Grade 3 view
2. Anterior airway, unable to angle ETT directly toward the vocal cords during direct laryngoscopy or with Glidescope

Equipment

1. Blade
2. ETT
3. Bougie
4. Second provider
5. +/– Magill forceps (Fig. 13.1)

© The Author(s), under exclusive license to Springer Nature Switzerland AG 2021
C. Sampankanpanich Soria et al., *Anesthesiology Resident Manual of Procedures*,
https://doi.org/10.1007/978-3-030-65732-1_13

Fig. 13.1 In some situations, it may be difficult to advance a Bougie under direct laryngoscopy with your own hand. If a Magill forceps is available (usually available in code bags and anesthesia cart), you can direct laryngoscopy (DL) with your left hand and use your right hand to hold the Magill forceps, grasp the Bougie, and then advance the Bougie. The Magill provides better control over the Bougie and allows you to grasp it more distally for better maneuverability. Remember that Magill forceps easily tear tissue and cause bleeding. Keep them closed until you're touching the object you intend to grasp

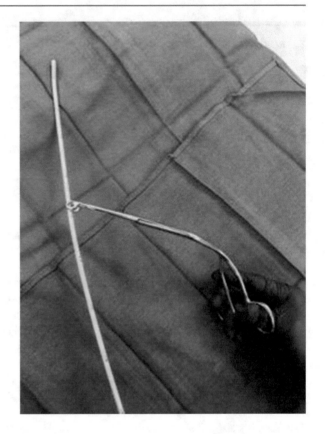

Instructions

1. Optimize patient positioning (room for head extension, tragus in line with sternum, flat chest).
2. Perform direct laryngoscopy.
3. Hold blade in place and maintain best view.
   (a) Tip: To prevent fatigue, tuck your left elbow into your left side and push your weight forward to lift the blade up.
4. Do not take your eyes off of your view (cords, epiglottis, corniculate cartilages).
5. Second provider places the Bougie in your right hand with the crook distal and facing anteriorly. Wrapping the front portion of the Bougie around your finger or using your fingertips to create a hockey stick bend at the distal end immediately prior to use helps to obtain proper shape at the tip to enter trachea blindly after passing beneath epiglottis.
6. Insert the Bougie underneath the epiglottis.
7. Feel the crook of the Bougie hit the tracheal rings.

8. If there is difficulty angling the Bougie anteriorly toward the cords, angle Bougie in the corner of the patient's mouth on the right side. Use this as a lever to lift the distal end of the Bougie up.
9. If still unable to angle upward, let the Bougie sit in the oropharynx.
10. Take the Magill forceps and grasp the Bougie distally and use the forceps to reach deeper into the oropharynx and push the Bougie past the cords.
11. You hold the Bougie in place between the cords and maintain best view with laryngoscopy; this allows for easier passage of ETT later.
12. Second provider slides the ETT over the Bougie. You then change hands – you hold onto the ETT and advance the ETT over the Bougie with a counterclockwise rotation to move past the arytenoid cartilage. The second provider holds onto the Bougie proximally to ensure it does not dislodge from the trachea.
13. You now hold onto the ETT.
14. Second provider gently removes the Bougie.
15. Verify ETT placement.
16. Secure ETT.

Intubating with C-Spine Precautions

14

Scenarios

1. Assumed unstable cervical spine
   (a) Trauma patient
   (b) Unable to clear patient due to mental status or distracting injury
2. Known unstable cervical spine
3. Severe cervical stenosis on MRI or any symptomatic cervical stenosis
4. Atlantoaxial instability (e.g., can be associated w/rheumatoid arthritis, trisomy 21)

Airway Management Decisions

1. Caution that airway manipulation in an unstable cervical spine can lead to cervical injury.
2. Goals
   (a) Maintain adequate spinal cord perfusion.
   (b) Avoid transection or direct physical damage to the spinal cord.
3. For trauma patients in particular, when planning airway management, consider possibility of secondary neurologic injury and anticipate how to protect the spinal cord.
4. Is the patient symptomatic with neck movement?
   (a) Numbness and weakness in upper extremities
   (b) Dizziness, syncope (vertebral artery symptoms?)
5. What does the imaging show?
   (a) MRI, CT C-spine
   (b) Spinal cord signaling changes, edema, stenosis, impingement
6. Intubate with or without C-collar? (see below)

© The Author(s), under exclusive license to Springer Nature Switzerland AG 2021
C. Sampankanpanich Soria et al., *Anesthesiology Resident Manual of Procedures*,
https://doi.org/10.1007/978-3-030-65732-1_14

7. Direct laryngoscopy? Glidescope? Fiberoptic bronchoscopy?
8. Asleep or awake?
   (a) Awake patient can protect his neck if the provider moves it in an inappropriate position.
   (b) After intubation, awake patient can undergo neurologic exam.
   (c) Caution with awake intubation: airway must be anesthetized well (topicalization or nerve blocks with local anesthetics) or supplemental sedation provided. Coughing can also cause significant neck movement and risk spinal cord injury.

How to Prevent Damage?

1. Maintain appropriate perfusion pressures intraoperatively.
2. Keep the neck in a neutral position to be able to maintain perfusion.
3. Discuss airway choice with the surgeon.
4. Everything is a spectrum.
   (a) Glidescope and even LMA placement can displace the c-spine just as much as direct laryngoscopy in some cases. Whatever technique you're using, you have to be aware of any manipulation that might translate to c-spine movement. Do the minimum necessary to obtain enough of a glottic view to intubate. Do not fight to get a grade 1 view when you don't really need it.
   (b) Mask ventilation can also be problematic if jaw thrust or head extension is inadvertently applied.

Intubating with C-Collar Still in Place

Pros
1. Don't need to replace C-collar when done with intubation.
2. Mechanical reinforcement to prevent you from manipulating airway too much.
3. Don't need a second provider for manual in line stabilization.
4. Using a Miller 3 blade may be helpful in this situation as it has less of a curve than the Macintosh. The extra length of the Miller blade overcomes some of the geometrical shortcomings of leaving the c-collar in place. However, this technique is awkward for inexperienced providers and should be practiced in advance.

Cons
1. Limited mouth opening: chin hits the anterior portion of C-collar.

Intubating Without C-Collar

Pros
1. More room for mouth opening.
2. Assistance from surgeon to ensure safe airway manipulation.

Instructions
1. Position patient for intubation:
   (a) Trauma bay patients all have C-collars. Trauma bay tables are flat, cannot be adjusted.
   (b) Technically not allowed to put patient in sniffing position because of head extension.
   (c) If in OR, ICU, or floor, can elevate head of bed to optimize positioning without extending neck.
2. After induction when patient will no longer move, ask the surgeon to remove the anterior portion of the cervical collar.
3. The surgeon then holds manual in-line stabilization.
4. Document who provided manual in-line stabilization.
5. Document that you performed gentle technique with manual in-line stabilization.

Intubating with Video Laryngoscope

15

Challenges

1. Get a grade 1 view of the vocal cords, and unable to angle the ETT/stylette anterior enough to reach it.
2. Unable to insert video laryngoscope due to limited mouth opening.
3. Unable to insert ETT because video laryngoscope takes up too much room in the oropharynx.

Equipment

1. Video laryngoscope with appropriate size blade, usually Mac 3 for adults.
2. Appropriate sized ETT, usually 7.0 or 8.0 ETT.
3. Surgical lubricant.

Instructions

1. Turn on the Video laryngoscope at least a few minutes prior to use.
   (a) Warm video laryngoscope + warm oropharynx = no fogging.
   (b) Cold video laryngoscope + warm oropharynx = fogging = bad view.
2. Optimize patient positioning (room for head extension, tragus in line with sternum, flat chest).
3. Lubricate video laryngoscope stylette generously and run through ETT a couple times to ensure moves smoothly.
4. Video laryngoscope insertion: straight down midline with a tongue sweep to left.
5. Hold ETT at proximal end to provide greater maneuverability.
   (a) Small movements proximally = greater movements distally

© The Author(s), under exclusive license to Springer Nature Switzerland AG 2021
C. Sampankanpanich Soria et al., *Anesthesiology Resident Manual of Procedures*,
https://doi.org/10.1007/978-3-030-65732-1_15

6. Do not lift the video laryngoscope too much, as this can distort the anatomy of the oropharynx and make it difficult to pass the ETT. Do not need a full view of the entire cords.
7. Once you've advanced the ETT tip to the epiglottis, push the ETT off of stylette and into trachea using your right thumb. This maneuver requires some grip repositioning.
8. As you advance the ETT through the cords, make a counterclockwise twisting motion so that ETT does not get stuck on the arytenoids.
9. Advance ETT cuff 1–2 cm past the vocal cords.
10. Second provider removes stylette while you watch the ETT remain in place between the vocal cords.
11. Then finally remove the video laryngoscope and secure ETT.

Intubating on the Ground

16

Scenarios

1. Patient found down in pharmacy, hospital lobby, bathroom, courtyard, etc.
2. No gurney or bed nearby to relocate patient.
3. Patient morbidly obese, unable to lift him to a bed.

Intubating Positions

Still try to optimize sniffing position as much as possible (room for head extension, tragus in line with sternum, and flat chest). Use towels/blankets/pillows to create shoulder roll.

#1 Sniper

Contraindications
1. You are pregnant.
2. Not enough room for you to lie down on the floor.

Technique
1. You lie flat on your stomach and rest your elbows on the ground.
2. Direct laryngoscopy with left hand.

Challenges
1. Rely on upper arm and abdominal strength to lift on direct laryngoscopy.
2. Unable to use body weight mechanics / angles because you are lying flat on the ground.

C. Sampankanpanich Soria et al., *Anesthesiology Resident Manual of Procedures*,
https://doi.org/10.1007/978-3-030-65732-1_16

#2 Toddler

Contraindications
1. No room at head of patient (e.g., blocked in a corner).

Technique
1. You sit on your buttocks with your legs extended out to your sides. The patient's head is directly in front of you.
2. Direct laryngoscopy with left hand.

Challenges
1. Rely on upper arm and abdominal strength to lift on direct laryngoscopy.
2. Unable to use body weight mechanics / angles because you are sitting on floor.

#3 Kneeling

Contraindications
1. No room at head of patient.

Technique
1. You kneel at patient's head and crouch down to look into mouth.
2. Direct laryngoscopy with left hand.

Challenges
1. Your view is relatively high up. Must crouch down to look into mouth.

#4 Reverse Direct Laryngoscopy

Utility
1. Only option when you cannot position yourself at the head of the patient traditionally.
2. Patient has their head in a corner of the room.
3. Patient in orthopedic surgery frame and unable to remove bed frame.

Technique
1. You position yourself at the patient's right side.
2. Scissor the mouth open with your left hand.
3. Direct laryngoscopy with your right hand.
4. Lean forward to look into the mouth to see view.
5. Insert endotracheal tube with your left hand.

Challenges
1. Reverse positioning from what you are accustomed to.

Double-Lumen Endotracheal Tubes

17

Indications for One-Lung Ventilation

Choosing a Double-Lumen Endotracheal Tube

Why Use a Double-Lumen Endotracheal Tube

Equipment

1. Appropriate-sized Double-Lumen Tube (DLT), usually left-sided (Table 17.1)/ (Table 17.2)/(Table 17.3)
2. One size up and one size down DLT (available in OR, keep in sterile packaging)
3. Fiberoptic bronchoscope – ideally large size, verify depending on size of DLT
4. Silicone lubricant for bronchoscope
5. Surgilube or lidocaine ointment to coat outside of DLT
6. Clamps to block tube lumens as needed
7. Adaptors to connect DLT to ventilator circuit
8. Nasal cannula
9. Mapleson bag attached to auxiliary oxygen port
10. French suction catheter

Table 17.1 List of absolute, relative (strong), and relative (weak) indications for using one-lung ventilation

Absolute	Protective isolation	Massive hemorrhage
		Infection
	Unilateral lung lavage	Aspiration
		Pulmonary contusion
		Pneumonia
		Unilateral pulmonary edema
	Video-Assisted Thoracoscopic Surgery	
	Control of ventilation distribution	Bronchopleural fistula or bronchocutaneous fistula
		Giant cyst or bullae
		Major bronchial disruption or trauma
		Differential ventilation (e.g., single lung transplant)
Relative (strong)	Surgical exposure	
	Thoracic aortic aneurysm	
	Pneumonectomy	
	Upper lobectomy	
Relative (weak)	Esophageal surgery	
	Middle and lower lobectomy	
	Thoracoscopy under general anesthesia	

Table 17.2 Comparing sizing of double-lumen endotracheal tubes in men versus women, and indications for placement or right- versus left-sided double-lumen endotracheal tubes

Size	Men	Women
	39–41 Fr	37–39 Fr
	Based on height	
Side	Right	Left
	Intubate the right mainstem bronchus, aperture similar to Murphy eye to facilitate ventilation of RUL	Intubate the left mainstem bronchus
	Less common, harder to place: sharp takeoff of R mainstem bronchus	More common, harder to place
	Indications: left pneumonectomy, surgery on left bronchus	

Table 17.3 Comparison of advantages and disadvantages to using a double-lumen endotracheal tube

Advantages	Disadvantages
Completely isolate one lung to ventilate	Difficult to place, large size
Can ventilate the isolated lung	Challenging, especially if patient has a difficult airway
Can add PEEP/CPAP when oxygenation is a problem on one-lung ventilation	At end of case, if remaining intubated, must exchange DLT for single-lumen ETT: challenging with airway edema, difficult intubation on first attempt, etc.
	Cannot target a specific lobe
	Can dislodge during case with patient repositioning

How to Place a DLT – Assuming Left-Sided DLT

1. Perform preoperative airway exam. If difficult intubation is anticipated, set up video laryngoscope and/or bronchoscope in anticipation of poor view with direct laryngoscopy.
2. Set up fiberoptic bronchoscope to verify appropriate positioning after intubation.
3. Assemble double-lumen tube: ETT, stylette, and 15 mm adaptors on the tracheal part and the bronchial part of the ETT.
4. Lubricate stylette and outside of ETT well.
   (a) Consider using lidocaine ointment instead of surgilube.
5. Curve the tip of the tube anteriorly to assist with placement, essentially 90 degrees counterclockwise to what will be the DLT final position. Even with a grade 1 view, the ETT tends to dip down into the esophagus.
6. Optimize patient positioning for intubation (tragus in line with sternum, room for head extension, and flat chest).
7. Perform direct laryngoscopy.
8. Insert double-lumen ETT.
   (a) Choke up on the double-lumen ETT. Small maneuvers proximally equal larger movements distally.
   (b) Lubricated ETT slides more easily past vocal cords.
9. If you are having trouble inserting the DLT using direct laryngoscopy, use the video laryngoscope.
10. Once DLT is inserted:
    (a) Remove stylette.
    (b) Inflate both cuffs (less air in bronchial cuff than tracheal cuff).
    (c) Connect tracheal tube and bronchial tube parts to their adaptors (between 15 mm adaptor and circuit; right-angled; has port to insert scope or suction catheter).
    (d) Confirm appropriate $ETCO_2$ capnogram.
11. Insert fiberoptic bronchoscope down the tracheal lumen of the DLT.
    (a) Confirm that the tracheal lumen opens just above the carina.
    (b) Confirm RUL takeoff: the only lobe to have three orifices (but can be fooled).
    (c) Confirm that you can see the blue bronchial cuff distally in the left mainstem bronchus.
12. Remove FOB scope from the tracheal lumen.
13. Now insert the FOB scope down the bronchial lumen of the DLT.
    (a) Confirm that the bronchial lumen opens into the left mainstem bronchus.
14. Remove bronchoscope.
15. Verify appropriate breath sounds with clamping and unclamping the bronchial and tracheal lumens.
16. Keep bronchoscope available in the OR in case double-lumen ETT positioning needs to be checked again during surgery.
17. Resume ventilation.

How to Use DLT for One-Lung Ventilation (Assuming Left-Sided DLT)

1. Ask surgeons when they would like you to drop the operative lung.
2. Ensure appropriate placement of DLT, especially with positioning changes (e.g., turning supine to lateral).
3. Verify that both bronchial and tracheal cuffs are inflated.
4. Confirm which side lung you need to deflate.
5. To deflate right lung:
   (a) Clamp the adaptor leading to the tracheal lumen (Fig. 17.1).
   (b) Open the suction port to the tracheal lumen.
   (c) Consider applying suction to the lumen to more rapidly deflate lung.
6. To deflate left lung:
   (a) Clamp the adaptor to the bronchial lumen.
   (b) Open the port to the bronchial lumen.
   (c) Consider applying suction to the lumen to more rapidly deflate lung.
7. Decrease tidal volumes (e.g., if normal TV is 600 cc with two lung ventilation, decrease to ~400 cc for one-lung ventilation and evaluate peak pressures and adequacy of ventilation).
8. To speed lung deflation:
   (a) Pass a 12–14 French suction catheter down the lumen of the operative lung, and maintain suction for 1–2 min.

How Does the Operative Lung Deflate?

Passive Deflation (Table 17.3 and Fig. 17.1)
1. Lack of supplemental oxygen being provided to alveoli.
2. Consumption of alveolar O_2 with time.

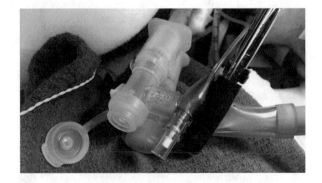

Fig. 17.1 Demonstration of how to use padded clamps to occlude one side of a double-lumen endotracheal tube when performing one-lung ventilation

Common DLT Malpositioning Errors

1. Entrance into the opposite bronchus to that intended (opposite lung will collapse).
2. Too deep in the bronchus (diminished breath sounds contralaterally).
3. Under-insertion (no breath sounds when tracheal lumen is used, as the endobronchial cuff is still sitting in the trachea).
4. Right-sided DLT occludes the RUL takeoff.

Emergency Cricothyroidotomy

18

Knife-Finger-Bougie

Pros
1. Fast
2. Simple
3. Minimal equipment
    (a) Scalpel should be readily available, ideally in code cart.
    (b) All other mandatory equipment is in the anesthesia code bag traditionally.

Equipment Needed
1. Chlorhexidine or iodine prep
2. Shoulder roll
3. Sterile gloves
4. Face mask and eye protection
5. Scalpel
6. Bougie
7. 6.0 ETT
8. Suture
9. +/− Marking pen

Instructions
1. Scenario: cannot intubate, cannot ventilate, no surgeon available immediately.
2. Call for help. Call for ENT / trauma surgeon / general surgeon to come STAT.
3. Optimize patient positioning: head extension to bring trachea anteriorly and stretch structures of neck to facilitate procedure.
    (a) Horizontal shoulder roll.
4. Stand at patient's side.
5. Palpate cricoid and thyroid cartilages. Identify midline.
    (a) If there is time, label anatomic structures with a marking pen.

© The Author(s), under exclusive license to Springer Nature Switzerland AG 2021
C. Sampankanpanich Soria et al., *Anesthesiology Resident Manual of Procedures*,
https://doi.org/10.1007/978-3-030-65732-1_18

6. With your left hand, grasp the cricoid cartilage/larynx with your thumb on the right side of the neck, and your 3rd/4th/5th digits on the left side of the neck.
7. Place your left index finger over the cricothyroid membrane, pointing inferiorly.
8. Take your scalpel with your right hand and choke up on it, holding close to the blade (Fig. 18.1).
9. Make a vertical incision 4 cm to cut into skin, subcutaneous tissue, and muscle.
   (a) The goal is to only have to make one incision. Do not want to waste time making multiple strokes to get through all the layers.
10. Use your left index finger to blunt dissect the tissue and find the cricothyroid membrane.
11. With the scalpel, now make a horizontal cut ~1 inch into the trachea (Fig. 18.1).
    (a) This is bloody.
    (b) Blood may spurt; make sure you are wearing protective face and eye equipment.
12. Put your left index finger into the trachea to extend the membrane.
    (a) Do not let go. Do not want to lose access.
13. Put the scalpel down.
14. Have a second provider hand you the Bougie.
15. With your right hand, insert the Bougie. Pass the Bougie alongside your left index finger and into the trachea (Fig. 18.2)/(Fig. 18.3).

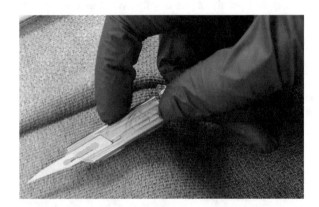

Fig. 18.1 Demonstration of how to hold the scalpel/blade. The goal is to make it through the skin, subcutaneous tissues, and muscle layers all in one stroke. Do not waste time making multiple strokes to reach the cricothyroid membrane. Time is critical

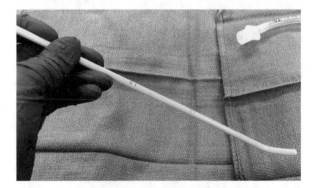

Fig. 18.2 After the cricothyroid membrane is cut and entry is established with either forceps or the provider's own finger(s), the Bougie is inserted

Fig. 18.3 The ETT is then inserted over the Bougie, using it as a conduit, and into the trachea

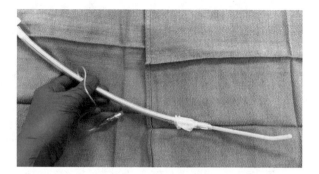

16. Switch to holding the Bougie with your left hand. Stabilize your left hand against the neck.
17. With your right hand, slide a 6.0 ETT over the Bougie until the cuff is just inside the trachea and no longer visible.
    (a) Do not advance further, as there is risk of mainstem intubation.
18. Remove the Bougie.
19. Inflate the cuff and test ventilation.
20. Secure ETT.

Complications
1. Failure
2. Bleeding
3. Infection
4. Damage to local structures: larynx, vessels, nerves, esophagus, cartilage, muscles
5. Cricoid fracture
6. Fistula formation
7. Scarring
8. Hypoxia
9. Death

Percutaneous Cricothyroidotomy

Cons
1. Kit not routinely available in anesthesia code bag

Equipment
1. Percutaneous cricothyroidotomy kit
    (a) Introducer needle and syringe
    (b) Guidewire
    (c) Dilator
    (d) Tracheostomy tube

2. Chloraprep stick
3. Shoulder roll
4. Sterile gloves
5. Face mask and eye protection
6. Marking pen

Instructions
1. Scenario: cannot intubate, cannot ventilate, no surgeon available immediately.
2. Call for help. Call for ENT / trauma surgeon / general surgeon to come STAT.
3. Optimize patient positioning: head extension to bring trachea anteriorly and stretch structures of neck to facilitate procedure.
   (a) Horizontal shoulder roll
4. Remember: this is Seldinger technique.
5. Palpate cricoid and thyroid cartilages. Identify midline.
   (a) If there is time, label anatomic structures with a marking pen.
   (b) Identify cricothyroid membrane.
6. Insert introducer needle and syringe at 90 degree angle to skin. Pull back on the syringe as you enter so you do not accidentally go through and through the trachea.
7. Once you draw back air, flatten the needle (aiming tip of needle caudad) and ensure you continue drawing back air.
8. Hold the needle with your left hand. Stabilize your left hand against the patient's neck.
9. Use your right hand to carefully disconnect the syringe from the needle.
10. Use your right hand to advance the guidewire through the needle.
11. Remove the needle and hold the guidewire with your left hand.
12. Use scalpel to make a vertical incision into skin, subcutaneous tissue, muscle, and cricothyroid membrane.
13. Advance the trach tube with dilator with the curved angle down, pointing towards the patient's feet.
14. Slide the dilator out and advance the trach tube.
15. Secure tube.

Laryngeal Mask Airways (LMAs)

19

Absolute Contraindications

1. Full stomach/significant aspiration risk
   - (a) Pregnant
   - (b) Obese
   - (c) Diabetic gastroparesis
   - (d) Inadequate NPO status
   - (e) Hiatal hernia
   - (f) Significant GERD
   - (g) Intestinal obstruction
2. Morbidly obese patients (non-rescue situations)
   - (a) Oropharyngeal adipose makes difficult proper placement of LMA and difficulty ventilating due to "restrictive" pulmonary parameters
3. Oropharyngeal pathology likely to result in poor mask fit
   - (a) For example, radiation therapy of hypopharynx/larynx, oropharyngeal masses
4. Glottic surgery where direct access to glottis is necessary

Relative Contraindications

1. Very long cases
   - (a) Not an exact cutoff, usually 2.5–3 h, very provider dependent
2. Prone position
   - (a) Provider comfort regarding prone, lateral, table turned 180 positioning and ability to troubleshoot LMA or intubate if LMA stops functioning

© The Author(s), under exclusive license to Springer Nature Switzerland AG 2021
C. Sampankanpanich Soria et al., *Anesthesiology Resident Manual of Procedures*,
https://doi.org/10.1007/978-3-030-65732-1_19

Indications

1. Short duration of case, and generally no muscle relaxation required, though some providers use with paralysis.
2. Minimize airway manipulation to decrease risk of bronchospasm, laryngo-spasm, etc.
   (a) Severe asthma, COPD
3. Rescue airway in cannot intubate, cannot ventilate situation.

Choosing an LMA

Table 19.1 Comparison of pros and cons of common types of laryngeal mask airways (LMAs)

LMA type	Pros	Cons
LMA Classic	"Routine use" LMA Full line of pediatric sizes Good seal Possibly less sore throat	Consider using purpose-designed LMAs for intubation
LMA Unique	Single use Disposable	Can make intubation easier if tube is cut Need a lot of lubrication to pass a standard ETT through lumen, OR use a narrower nasal RAE or micro-laryngoscopy ETT
LMA ProSeal	Softer silicone, less throat irritation/stimulation, but tends to fold over in larynx more often More likely than LMA classic to seal at airway pressures >20 cmH$_2$O, up to 30 cmH$_2$O Theoretically tighter seal against glottis opening w/o increasing mucosal pressure Better for positive pressure ventilation OG tube channel to decompress stomach	Cannot intubate through with standard fiberoptic technique (smaller lumen) Aintree catheter can assist with intubation if necessary
LMA Flexible	Suitable for head and neck procedures Airway tube can be positioned away from surgical field without loss of seal Flexible stem reduces tension from breathing circuit Wire-reinforced tube resists kinking and cuff dislodgement	Can be difficult to place due to flimsiness of tube Not an ideal intubation conduit (smaller lumen)
LMA Cookgas	Firm, stiff, may be more likely to cause sore throat Better as rescue, emergency resource rather than routine use Best intubation conduit Easily removable adaptor, short wide shaft Wide enough lumen to easily intubate through	

Table 19.1 (continued)

LMA type	Pros	Cons
LMA Fastrach	Rigid, anatomically curved tube Wide enough to accept an 8.0 ETT Short enough to ensure passage beyond the vocal cords Rigid handle for one-handed insertion/removal/adjustment Epiglottic elevating bar in mask aperture Ramp that directs ETT centrally and anteriorly to reduce risk of arytenoid trauma or esophageal placement Can facilitate blind intubation	Must have specialized parts ETT adaptor difficult to remove
LMA Supreme	Follows natural curvature of the oropharynx so goes in smoothly Stiff handle, easy insertion Channel to pass orogastric tube to suction stomach Bite block built in	Cannot intubate through (smaller lumen diameter) Aintree catheter can facilitate intubation

Instructions

1. Preparation of the LMA (Table 19.1)
   (a) One nickel's worth of surgical lubricant or lidocaine ointment over the exterior surface of the LMA bowl, which will slide posteriorly down the larynx.
   (b) Consider adding 10–15 cc of air to the LMA or leave as is.
2. Back-up airway equipment (Table 19.2)
   (a) Always have a laryngoscope, ETT, and succinylcholine (unless contraindicated, then rocuronium).
   (b) Indications for emergency intubation: laryngospasm, unable to seat LMA, surgical emergency.
3. Induction
   (a) Optimize patient positioning (tragus in line with sternum, room for head extension, flat chest).
   (b) Administer induction agents of choice.
   (c) Recommend minimizing fentanyl use until after inserting LMA and getting patient to spontaneous ventilate.
4. confirm patient is deep enough for LMA placement
   (a) Eyelid/lash reflex
   (b) Mandible feels loose
5. Techniques for LMA insertion
   (a) Fingers in mouth (not really recommended but commonly done)
       (i) Tilt head back to optimize head extension.
       (ii) Scissor the mouth open with your right hand on the molars.

(iii) With your left hand, insert the LMA straight down, perpendicular to the floor.

(iv) If met with resistance, push down on the LMA tube with your left hand while using your right fingers (or tongue depressor, see below) to guide the LMA bowl down the oropharynx and larynx.

(v) Caution: if you plan to put your fingers in the patient's mouth, make sure you double glove and ensure the patient is deeply anesthetized. Otherwise, you will cut your hands on the patient's teeth and/or the patient will bite you.

(b) Thumb to chin

(i) Tilt head back to optimize head extension.

(ii) Use your left thumb to pull down the patient's chin.

(iii) With your right hand, insert the LMA straight down, perpendicular to the floor.

(iv) If met with resistance, push down on the LMA tube with your left hand while using your right fingers (or tongue depressor, see below) to guide the LMA bowl down the oropharynx and larynx.

(c) Scissor, tongue blade

(i) Tilt head back to optimize head extension.

(ii) Scissor the mouth open with your right hand on the molars.

(iii) With your left hand, use the tongue blade to push the tongue anteriorly and open space in the oropharynx.

(iv) With your right hand, insert the LMA straight down, perpendicular to the floor.

(d) Scissor, direct laryngoscopy

(i) Direct laryngoscopy as you normally would to intubate, then insert the LMA with your right hand. It helps to have tongue fully swept to left and laryngoscope perhaps a bit to the left of midline if possible. Deflating the LMA can provide more room for it to pass the oropharyngeal entrance if size is an issue.

(e) Deflate and twist

(i) Deflate the LMA completely.

(ii) Tilt head back to optimize head extension.

(iii) Open the mouth with thumb to push chin down.

(iv) Insert the LMA straight down, perpendicular to floor, with bowl facing towards you.

(v) Once the tip of the LMA is likely at the base of the tongue and just encountering the posterior pharynx, twist the LMA 180 degrees so the bowl faces anteriorly. Inflate LMA.

6. Connect LMA to circuit. Confirm appropriate placement via $ETCO_2$ capnogram.

7. Check LMA seal pressure:

(a) Close APL valve to $10 \rightarrow 15 \rightarrow 20 \rightarrow 25$ cmH$_2$O to detect a leak.

(b) Ideal seal pressure of 20 cmH$_2$O: ensures that LMA will not be dislodged at such a peak pressure.

8. Secure LMA.

9. Place patient on volatile anesthetics. Avoid nitrous oxide to decrease risk of gastric distension and micro-aspirations. Is there good data for this? This is the type of thing where if you have data you should reference it, if it is at the level of an opinion then qualify with something like "some practitioners."
10. Maintain spontaneous ventilation, or pressure support ventilation for some support.
11. Titrate fentanyl to respiratory rate.

Troubleshooting LMAs

Table 19.2 List of common complications that occur when using LMAs, and techniques to troubleshoot such challenges

Scenario	Complications	Treatment	
Inadequate anesthesia	Coughing, breath holding Laryngospasm Coughing/bucking → dislodged LMA	Deepen with propofol Increase volatile anesthetic Troubleshoot LMA placement	
Deflated LMA	LMA bowl folds on itself, obstructing passage of airflow	Add air to LMA and reposition May require bilateral jaw thrust, manipulation to help seat properly	
Stiff mouth opening	Not enough room to even insert LMA into the oropharynx	Scissor mouth open with fingers on molars Tongue blade to elevate tongue Thumb to pull down chin	
Low tidal volumes Unable to ventilate Loss of ETCO$_2$ capnogram	LMA obstructing airflow LMA poorly seated LMA dislodged (light patient, manipulation of head/neck by surgeon) Laryngospasm	Initial maneuvers:	Notify surgeons. Call for help if needed. Increase to 100% FiO2. Try to manually hand ventilate the patient.
		If unable to hand ventilate via LMA:	Try to manipulate LMA by jaw thrust, adjustment of tube. Goal is to help lift the tongue/epiglottis anteriorly off of the posterior pharyngeal wall If still unsuccessful, remove LMA completely
		After removing LMA, mask ventilate:	Ensure you are able to mask ventilate (chin lift, jaw thrust, airway adjuncts, two-handed technique)
		If able to mask ventilate:	Re-attempt LMA placement If successful, proceed with case If unsuccessful, consider intubation
		If unable to mask ventilate:	Low threshold for laryngospasm Treat with positive pressure breaths, or propofol and/or succinylcholine to break laryngospasm Consider emergency intubation if needed

Troubleshooting Tracheostomies

20

Things to Know About a Patient's Existing Tracheostomy Tube

Multiple Purposes of a Tracheostomy Tube

Common Complications of a Tracheostomy Tube

Airway and Breathing Assessment in a Patient with a Tracheostomy Tube Who Has Arrested

Ventilation and Reintubation After Removal of Tracheostomy Tube

Components of a Tracheostomy Tube

Faceplate (aka neck flange): where the ties or sutures are connected to secure the tracheostomy tube; this is where you will find what kind of trach tube the patient has (number 4.0, 6.0, etc.) and the dimensions of the tube (cuffed, uncuffed; fenestrated, unfenestrated; XL).

Outer cannula: the main body of the tube that is inserted into the trachea; a single cannula tube = 1 cannula only; a double cannula tube = outer cannula + inner cannula.

Inner cannula: dual cannula tube = outer cannula + inner cannula; inner cannula can be removed for cleaning or be replaced to help managed secretions; with a dual cannula tube, you need the inner cannula to connect to breathing circuit.

© The Author(s), under exclusive license to Springer Nature Switzerland AG 2021
C. Sampankanpanich Soria et al., *Anesthesiology Resident Manual of Procedures*,
https://doi.org/10.1007/978-3-030-65732-1_20

Shaft: standard adult tracheostomy tubes are 75 mm in length; some necks are thicker in diameter; longer tracheostomy tubes are available (XL = extended length, proximally or distally).

Cuff: blocks the airway when inflated by way of inflation line for patients who require ventilation or have poor swallowing ability; presence of pilot balloon outside indicates whether or not the trach has a cuff, and if the cuff is inflated.

Obturator: aka pilot; assists with insertion of tracheostomy tube; inner cannula is removed and obturator is inserted; has blunt tip and cushions the placement of the tube into the trachea to avoid tissue damage; immediately following placement, the obturator is removed and replaced with the inner cannula.

How to Change Out an Existing Tracheostomy Tube in an Awake Patient

1. Baseline information should be obtained about the indications for and type of tracheostomy tube (Table 20.1)/(Table 20.2).
2. Attempts should be made to troubleshoot the tracheostomy tube and identify possible explanations for why the tracheostomy tube is not functioning properly (Table 20.3)/(Table 20.4).
3. If the decision has been made that the tracheostomy tube needs to be changed, it is best to do this in the safest environment possible. The safest environment is the operating room if at all possible, especially in less mature tracheostomies. If the patient is unstable and time is not permitting, this may need to be done in less optimal environments such as the intensive care unit or floor at bedside (Table 20.5).
4. Notify ENT and/or trauma surgery.
5. Goal: exchange an uncuffed tracheostomy tube for a tracheostomy tube. Bad things happen with uncuffed tubes under general anesthesia.
6. Psychological buy-in from the patient: talk to them, reassure them of what is going to happen.

Table 20.1 List of key pieces of information to obtain when troubleshooting tracheostomy tubes

Why does the patient have a tracheostomy?	Respiratory	Apnea
		Irregular respiratory pattern
		Spontaneous ventilation but requires assisted positive pressure ventilation
	Neurologic	Stroke
		Elevated ICP
		Traumatic brain injury
		Spinal cord injury
		Neuromuscular disorder, paralysis/ weakness
	Ear/nose/throat	Postoperative course after operation on trachea, larynx
		Abnormal airway anatomy

Table 20.1 (continued)

What type of tracheostomy does the patient have?	Size	Adults: 6.0, 7.0, 8.0	
	Length	Regular	
		Extended length	Anterior-posterior (e.g., obese patient) Cephalad-caudad (e.g., tall patient)
	Cuffed	Cuffed: will see a pilot balloon on the outside Un-cuffed: will leak with positive pressure ventilation Strongly recommend changing to cuffed ETT or trach, even if planning spontaneous ventilation. High risk of inability to ventilate if spontaneous ventilation is lost	
	Fenestrated	Purpose: allow speech. Air enters through trach, some air expelled through fenestration, past vocal cords, and out mouth, enabling speech Air will leak through nose and mouth Need non-fenestrated inner cannula to occlude the fenestrated openings of outer cannula	
	Double-cannulated	Outer cannula automatically remains in patient Most circuits only connect to the inner cannula Caution: not all patients have the inner cannula with them at bedside. In this case, a cannula from a fresh tracheostomy kit will be needed	
	Passy Muir valve	One-way valve, air goes into, not out of, the tracheostomy tube If accidentally try to ventilate with cuff inflated, will inflate lungs repeatedly without deflation → barotrauma, volutrauma Must deflate cuff for ventilation Not ideal for positive pressure ventilation	
	Obturator	Plastic or metal tube to maintain patent stoma Not intended for ventilation	
How old is the stoma?	<1 week	Not much granulation tissue If tracheostomy tube becomes dislodged, difficult to insert tube through young stoma; significant	
	>2–3 weeks	Granulation tissue well-formed Easier to reinsert tube through older stoma; less risk of creating false passage outside of the airway	

(continued)

Table 20.1 (continued)

What is the patient's airway anatomy?	Normal larynx		Anesthesiologist needs to know:
			1. Can this patient be mask ventilated?
	Abnormal larynx	Post-tracheal resection	2. Can this patient be intubated from above by direct laryngoscopy?
		Post-laryngectomy	3. Is the only access to the patient's trachea through the neck?
Are there any other devices associated with the tracheostomy?	Tracheo-esophageal piece		Enables speech
	Speaking valve		Warms air
	Humidifying device		Maintains stoma while patient ventilates
	Obturator		through nose and mouth

Table 20.2 Short-term and long-term explanations for why a patient has a tracheostomy tube

Temporary			Permanent	
Upper airway protection	Head/neck trauma		Long-term mechanical ventilation	Spinal cord injury
	Massive fluid resuscitation			Brain injury: stroke, ICH
	Burns			Neuromuscular disease
	Cannot intubate, cannot ventilate			Irreversible cause of apnea/ hypoventilation
	Emergency in OR or at bedside	Percutaneous (commonly done by pulmonologists, critical care)		Irreversible alteration to traditional airway anatomy (tracheal resection, laryngectomy)
		Slit type		
		Flap (more secure stoma)		
Weaning from mechanical ventilation	Predicted, limited duration of illness			

Table 20.3 Common complications that occur from in situ tracheostomy tubes based on how long the tracheostomy tube has been in place

Immediate	Hemorrhage
	Loss of airway (dislodged, unable to reinsert tracheostomy tube)
Short-term	Blockage (soft tissue, clot, secretions/mucus)
	Complete or partial tracheostomy tube displacement
Long-term	Tracheomalacia
	Tracheal stenosis
	Stoma problems related to healing
	Artificial airway devices: blocked, displaced

7. Pre-medication:
    (a) Midazolam 1–2 mg to relieve anxiety
    (b) Fentanyl 25–50 mcg to prevent coughing
    (c) Glycopyrrolate 0.1–0.2 mg to decrease airway secretions
8. Routine ASA monitors.

9. Positioning.
    (a) Vertical shoulder roll to extend the neck and shoulders
    (b) Moves trachea anterior
10. Simple face mask at 10 L/min for patient to breathe through nose/mouth.
11. Connect existing tracheostomy tube to ventilator circuit with a bronchoscopy elbow in place. Maintain spontaneous ventilation.
12. Insert fiberoptic bronchoscope. Topicalize airway with preservative free lidocaine while advancing the FOB scope. Assess the stoma and airway (e.g., granulation tissue, mucus, blood, obstruction).
13. If the trachea looks favorable, remove the FOB scope.
14. Numb the area around the stoma/existing tracheostomy tube.
    (a) 1–2% lidocaine in a syringe attached to a 25 G needle.
    (b) Tilt the tracheostomy tube to the side to create a crevice between the tube and the skin. Dribble local anesthetic into this area, an angiocatheter attached to syringe can facilitate this. Repeat circumferentially.
    (c) Goal is to prevent the patient from coughing out the new tube.
15. With an Aintree catheter over the FOB scope, insert into existing tracheostomy tube.
16. With the scope 2 cm proximal to the carina, slide the Aintree catheter over the FOB scope and remove the FOB scope.
17. Slide the old tracheostomy tube over the Aintree catheter and remove completely from the neck.

Table 20.4 Algorithm for assessing and managing non-functioning tracheostomy tubes

Initial survey	Call for help		Rapid response or code blue ENT, trauma/general surgery Fiberoptic bronchoscope		
	History		Why is the patient trached? Type of trach? Age of stoma? Current ENT anatomy? Trach-dependent? Difficult intubation?		
	Physical		Looks, listen, and feel		
Is the native airway patent?	NO	CANNOT intubate from nose or mouth	YES	Can mask ventilate	
		CANNOT mask ventilate		Can intubate through nose, mouth, or neck	
		Only airway access is through the neck			
Is the patient breathing?	NO	If patent airway, bag mask ventilate	YES	Apply supplemental oxygen to face and tracheostomy	
				Optimize patient positioning – shoulder roll, head of bed elevated	
		Assess tracheostomy patency		If patent airway, assistive maneuvers	Chin lift Jaw thrust Nasal trumpet Oral airway
				Assess tracheostomy patency	

(continued)

Table 20.4 (continued)

How do you assess tracheostomy patency?	Attach Mapleson circuit to tracheostomy tube	If patient is spontaneously ventilating, watch for bag movement If patient is apneic, apply small, gentle test breaths.[a] If resistance, stop immediately		
	Ancillary trach devices present?	Remove	Decannulation caps Obturators Speaking valves used incorrectly Humidifiers	
	Inner cannula present?	Remove Inspect for obstruction (blood clot, mucus plug) Clean before reinsertion		
	Can you pass a suction catheter?	NO	If resistance, stop immediately to avoid creating trauma or false passage Try repositioning angle of tracheostomy tube, it may just be opening against back wall of trachea due to angle of entry sometimes this is due to over inflation of cuff as well	YES	Tracheostomy tube is patent Suction Consider partial obstruction Further inspect with FOB if available Continue to ventilate via tracheostomy tube
	Deflate the cuff	Able to ventilate	Tracheostomy tube is partially obstructed or displaced Continue to ventilate via tracheostomy tube	Unable to ventilate	Remove the tracheostomy tube[b] Continue applying supplemental oxygen to face and stoma

[a]Hand ventilate with caution when diagnosing airway patency. Vigorous ventilation of a displaced tracheostomy tube will create subcutaneous emphysema, potentially causing rapid airway obstruction and worsening access to the neck. Aggressive hand ventilation for resuscitation should only be done after confirming a secure airway

[b]Providers may hesitate to remove a tracheostomy tube because the patient was a difficult intubation or tracheostomy tube placement. However, it is harmful and useless to keeping a non-functioning tracheostomy tube in a patient. Do not delay removal of a blocked or displaced tracheostomy tube if a patient is deteriorating. Note: if tube is in trachea but need replacement, use tube exchanger

18. Slide the new tracheostomy or endotracheal tube over the Aintree catheter and into the neck.
19. Remove the Aintree catheter while leaving the new tube in place.
20. Confirm ventilation through the new tube.
21. Secure the new tube.
    (a) Tracheostomy tube – comes with Velcro wrap
    (b) Endotracheal tube – use Tegaderms or suture in place

Table 20.5 Techniques for restoring ventilation and reintubating a patient after a tracheostomy tube has been removed

	Ventilation		Reintubation	
If the upper airway is patent	Mask ventilation of the face[a]	Chin lift	Oral intubation	Anticipate difficult intubation
		Jaw thrust		
		Nasal trumpet		Uncut ETT to advance past stoma
		Oral airway		
		Occlude the stoma with wet gauze/ tegaderm		
	Mask ventilation of the stoma[a]	Pediatric-sized face mask	Stoma intubation	Optimize patient positioning: vertical shoulder roll, arms and neck extended; positions trachea anterior
				Tracheostomy tube of equal or smaller size than original
		Pediatric-sized LMA		If previous tracheostomy tube was too short and lumen was occluded by soft tissue, consider using XL (extended length)
		Minimize leaks through nose and mouth	Usually 6.0 in adults	Regular ETT Laryngoflex ETT (follows natural curvature of neck, lower risk of right mainstem intubation)
		Insert LMA and occlude the proximal portion		Armored ETT (soft, flexible, follows neck curvature)
		Occlude the nose/ mouth with gauze/ tegaderm		Consider inserting conduit first: Aintree catheter, FOB scope, Bougie, airway exchange catheter
				Risk of trauma and creation of false passage when inserting devices blindly through stoma
If the upper airway is *not* patent	Cannot face mask ventilate		Mask ventilate the stoma[a] (see above)	
	Cannot intubate through nose or mouth		Intubate the stoma (see above)	
	No aspiration risk b/c no connection between trachea and esophagus		Assess the trachea and stoma with FOB ENT assistance	

[a]The goal is oxygenation and ventilation, not necessarily intubation. A secure airway via an endotracheal tube or a tracheostomy tube is ideal, but not mandatory. The primary benefit is decreased aspiration risk. Prioritize effective oxygenation and ventilation via masking until a secure airway is safely established. Effective mask ventilation and oxygenation buys time until better resources and staff are available (e.g., ENT surgeons, fiberoptic bronchoscope, OR staff)

Ultrasound-Guided Peripheral IVs 21

Equipment

1. Ultrasound machine with linear probe, gel lubricant
2. Angiocatheter of various lengths and lumen sizes (Fig. 21.1)
   (a) 1.25″
   (b) 3″
3. Tourniquet
4. Non-sterile gauze
5. Alcohol wipes
6. Saline flush and IV pigtail
7. +/− Guidewire

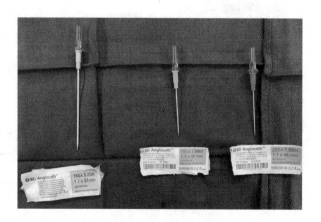

Fig. 21.1 Photograph of BD angiocatheters: (left) 16 G × 3.25 inch; (middle) 18 G × 1.88 inch; (right) 20 G × 1.88 inch

© The Author(s), under exclusive license to Springer Nature Switzerland AG 2021
C. Sampankanpanich Soria et al., *Anesthesiology Resident Manual of Procedures*,
https://doi.org/10.1007/978-3-030-65732-1_21

Instructions

1. Identify target site (e.g., basilic vein).
2. Place the tourniquet high, close to the axilla.
3. Position the patient's arm supine and externally rotated to expose the medial upper arm.
4. First identify the vein, scanning up and down to determine the length of the vein before branches take off. Trace the vein proximally and distally.
   (a) Common errors: trying to insert a catheter where there is a branch or valve. You will obtain flow but will not be able to thread the catheter past the valve or bifurcation.
5. Note the position of the brachial artery. Be careful to avoid the artery.
6. Determine the depth of the subcutaneous tissue to pass through.
   (a) Thin patients: a standard angiocatheter as used for arterial lines, 1.25″, is acceptable.
   (b) Short veins: use the shorter angiocatheter, 1.25″.
   (c) Edematous, obese patients: use a longer angiocatheter, 3″.
7. Determine approach to placement (see below).

Cross-Sectional View: Slide Catheter off Needle

1. With your left hand, hold the ultrasound probe with the beam perpendicular to path of vein.
2. Obtain cross-sectional view.
3. With your right hand, hold the angiocatheter like a pencil and insert at 30–45° angle.
4. Watch the tip of the needle enter the lumen of the vessel.
5. When the needle tip is in the lumen of the vessel (ideally the center), confirm blood flash in the catheter.
6. Flatten the angle of the needle.
7. Confirm continued blood flow.
8. Set aside the ultrasound probe.
9. Continue to hold the needle with your right hand.
10. Use your left hand to slide the catheter off of the needle and into the vein.
11. The catheter should slide smoothly. Do not force if there is resistance.

Cross-Sectional View: Advance-Needle Tip-Repeat

1. With your left hand, hold the ultrasound probe with the beam perpendicular to path of vein.
2. Obtain cross-sectional view.
3. With your right hand, hold the angiocatheter like a pencil and insert at 30–45° angle.
4. Watch the tip of the needle enter the lumen of the vessel.

5. Flatten the angle of the needle.
6. Move the ultrasound probe more proximally about 1–2 mm.
7. Advance the needle and watch the tip in the lumen.
8. Repeat steps 6 and 7 until most of the catheter is in the vessel.
9. Set aside the ultrasound probe.
10. Slide the catheter off of the needle and into the vessel.
11. Remove tourniquet, attach pigtail, and ensure it flushes easily.

Longitudinal View

1. With your left hand, hold the ultrasound probe with the beam parallel to the path of the vein.
2. Obtain longitudinal view.
3. With your right hand, hold the angiocatheter like a pencil and insert at a 30° angle.
4. Advance the needle tip into the lumen of the vein.
5. Flatten the needle, and advance the tip.
6. Visualize the tip advancing through the lumen, and adjust the angle as needed.
7. Once most of the catheter is in the vein, set aside the ultrasound probe.
8. Continue to hold the needle with your right hand.
9. Use your left hand to slide the remainder of the catheter off of the needle and into the vein.
10. Remove tourniquet, attach pigtail, and ensure it flushes easily.

Through and Through

1. Caveat: recommended as last resort due to risk of hematoma formation, not a foolproof technique, not ideal.
2. With your left hand, hold the ultrasound probe with the beam perpendicular to path of vein.
3. Obtain cross-sectional view.
4. With your right hand, hold the angiocatheter like a pencil and insert at 30–45° angle.
5. Watch the tip of the needle enter the lumen of the vessel.
6. Confirm flash in the catheter.
7. Maintain the angle, and advance the needle through past the other side of the vessel.
8. Set aside the ultrasound probe.
9. Switch hands to hold the catheter with your left hand.
10. Remove the needle with your right hand.
11. Slowly withdraw the catheter back until flow is obtained.
12. Thread the guidewire through the catheter into the vessel with your right hand.
13. Slide the catheter off of the guidewire and into the vessel with your left hand.
14. Remove tourniquet, attach pigtail, and ensure it flushes easily.

Where to Look for Peripheral IV

22

Scenario

1. No ultrasound available
2. Pediatrics patient
3. Edematous patient
4. Thick subcutaneous tissue
5. Dark skin
6. Unable to visualize veins

Sites to Look "Blindly"

1. "Intern vein:" lateral wrist/distal forearm
2. Anterior wrist: small, good for a 22 G PIV to induce patient. When asleep, one can look for larger vein
3. Anterior cubital fossa
4. Saphenous: relax the leg externally rotated at hips. Hold the distal foot down to bring the medial malleolus anterior. Insertion site is 1 cm anterior and 1 cm superior to the medial malleolus
5. Hand between 4th and 5th metacarpals
6. Hand between 3rd and 4th metacarpals
7. Also, don't forget to look at the external jugular, which is sometimes easily visible in patients who otherwise have no visible sites

Instructions

1. Insert needle at 45° angle.
2. Fan the needle in and out slowly medially and laterally.
3. When flash is seen, stop, flatten the needle, and advance 1–2 mm.
4. Thread the catheter off of the needle and into the vein.

© The Author(s), under exclusive license to Springer Nature Switzerland AG 2021
C. Sampankanpanich Soria et al., *Anesthesiology Resident Manual of Procedures*,
https://doi.org/10.1007/978-3-030-65732-1_22

Subclavian Central Lines without Ultrasound

23

Equipment

1. Central line kit
   - (a) Introducer needle and syringe
   - (b) Guidewire
   - (c) Manometry catheter and tubing
   - (d) Catheter (e.g., Cordis, double lumen, triple lumen)
   - (e) Scalpel
   - (f) Suture
2. Biopatch
3. Tegaderm
4. Sterile gauze
5. Sterile flushes
6. Caps for catheter (e.g., luer lock caps, stopcocks)

Choosing a Side

The following instructions assume left-sided placement (Table 23.1).

Table 23.1 Comparison of placing central lines in the right versus left intrajugular vein

Left	Right
More common site	Less common site
Straightest path from L subclavian vein to SVC	Steep angle from R subclavian vein to SVC
Guidewire less likely to cross up L IJ or to R innominate	Guidewire more likely to cross up R IJ or to L subclavian

© The Author(s), under exclusive license to Springer Nature Switzerland AG 2021
C. Sampankanpanich Soria et al., *Anesthesiology Resident Manual of Procedures*,
https://doi.org/10.1007/978-3-030-65732-1_23

Positioning

1. Roll up a blanket and tape together to ensure firm roll.
2. Place under patient's upper back, midline, vertically.
3. Extend the neck and relax the shoulders to the sides.
4. Opens up the patient's chest and positions the subclavian vein more superficially.
5. Provider stands at patient's left side, facing the patient.

Indications

1. Subclavian central lines are less commonly done.
2. Overall central lines are less commonly done without ultrasound.
3. Argument for better sterility of subclavian > internal jugular > femoral central lines.
4. Internal jugular central lines are contraindicated in neurosurgical cases or situations of elevated ICP, where IJ line placement may impede cerebral venous drainage.

Risks

1. Pneumothorax
   (a) Place patient on 100% FiO_2.
   (b) Decrease tidal volumes to decrease risk of pneumothorax during placement.
2. Bleeding
   (a) Subclavian vein and artery are anchored by soft tissues.
   (b) Hard to reach subclavian artery to apply pressure if accidentally puncture the subclavian artery.
3. Infection

Instructions: Without Ultrasound

1. Palpate for sternal notch and lateral end of clavicle.
2. Identify midline of clavicle.
3. Place left index and middle fingers at mid-clavicular line, 1 cm underneath the clavicle. This will be insertion site.
4. Hold introducer needle and syringe in right hand, with right fingers constantly pulling back on plunger.
5. Insert needle as flat as possible, <30° angle, aiming towards the sternal notch.
   (a) *Avoid the temptation to steepen the angle.*
   (b) *Steep angle = higher risk of pneumothorax.*
6. Use left index and middle fingers to push down on the needle and remind yourself to stay as flat as possible.

7. Advance until hit flash.
8. If hit bone, this is likely clavicle. Gradually walk off the bone, more medially and inferiorly, until enter the vein.
9. The subclavian artery is deep to the subclavian vein. Sometimes you may cross through the vein and hit artery. If this happens, pull back until have venous return.
10. Once flash is obtained, draw back on plunger and ensure continuous easy return of blood.
11. Gently disconnect the syringe from the introducer needle.
12. Ensure no pulsatile flow.
13. Smoothly thread guidewire through the introducer needle.
14. Remove introducer needle over the guidewire.
15. Advance manometry catheter over the guidewire.
16. Remove guidewire from the manometry catheter.
17. Gently connect manometry tubing to manometry catheter.
18. Hold the manometry tubing down to allow it to fill by gravity.
19. Once full, then elevate the tubing up. Should NOT see the tubing continue to fill up.
    (a) The height of the column is pressure in cmH_2O. Divide this height by 1.36 to convert to mmHg.*
20. Disconnect the manometry tubing.
21. Thread the guidewire through the manometry catheter.
22. Remove the manometry catheter.
23. Make a skin nick with the scalpel.
24. Advance the central line catheter (e.g., Cordis, double, or triple lumen) over the guidewire, in a twisting motion.
25. Remove the guidewire.
26. Attach flushes and ensure all ports draw back blood and flush easily.
27. Attach luer lock caps or stopcocks.
28. Secure central line with suture.
29. Secure with biopatch, tegaderm.

*Conversion factor: Mercury (Hg) is 13.6 times the density of water (H_2O), and 10 mm = 1 cm. To convert cmH_2O to mmHg, divide by 1.36.

Caution

1. Keep your needle as parallel to the ground as possible.
2. Do not steepen your needle to advance into the vein.
3. To find the vein, press down on the needle with your left index, middle, and ring fingers, to push deeper and walk off the bone.
4. When placing any central line, always watch the monitors carefully for PVCs, ectopic beats.
5. A patient with a left bundle branch block who develops right heart irritation and a right bundle branch block can develop complete heart block and asystole.

How to Straighten out the Guidewire

1. Usually the guidewire is inserted through the sheath and introducer.
2. Sometimes with multiple attempts or accidental removal, the guidewire becomes removed from the sheath and/or introducer.
3. The guidewire is composed of a coiled wire over a central wire core.
4. To straighten the J-wire with one hand, stabilize the proximal part of the guidewire with your palm and 3rd, 4th, and 5th fingers.
5. With your thumb and index finger tips, pinch the guidewire (about 5 cm proximal to the J-tip) and push out, stretching the guidewire. This will straighten the guidewire for insertion.

Internal Jugular Central Line Without Ultrasound

24

Choosing a Side

Position

- Supine.
- Trendelenburg position – head down – to enlarge the IJ vein.
- Head slightly turned to contralateral side to expose the IJ and help identify landmarks. Do not turn too much, as this will position the IJ directly over the carotid artery, increasing the risk of accidental carotid artery puncture (Table 24.1).
- Shoulder roll horizontally underneath the scapula to extend the neck.

Landmarks

1. Palpate the sternal notch and clavicle.
2. Palpate the carotid artery, which lies medial to the internal jugular vein.

Table 24.1 How to choose right versus left side for intrajugular vein central line placement

Right side	Left side
More commonly done, especially if planning to insert Swan-Ganz catheter	Less commonly done
Shorter and straighter path from R IJ to SVC and RA	Longer and more curved path from L IJ to SVC and RA. Guidewire more likely to cross to R subclavian or R IJ

© The Author(s), under exclusive license to Springer Nature Switzerland AG 2021
C. Sampankanpanich Soria et al., *Anesthesiology Resident Manual of Procedures*,
https://doi.org/10.1007/978-3-030-65732-1_24

3. Identify the sternal and clavicular heads of the sternocleidomastoid muscle.
   (a) The sternal head is proximal and lateral to the sternal notch. Rubbing your fingers along this muscle, it feels like a string, bounces.
   (b) Use a marking pen to label the landmarks.
4. Trace the two heads of the sternocleidomastoid muscle proximally to where they form a V. The apex of the V is the goal insertion site of your needle.

Instructions

1. Equipment: central line kit
   (a) Finder needle and syringe
   (b) Introducer needle and syringe
   (c) Guidewire
   (d) Manometry catheter and tubing
   (e) Catheter (e.g., Cordis, double lumen, triple lumen)
   (f) Scalpel
   (g) Suture
   (h) Biopatch
   (i) Tegaderm
   (j) Sterile gauze
   (k) Sterile flushes
   (l) Caps for catheter (e.g., luer lock caps, stopcocks)
2. Locate insertion site using landmarks (see above).
3. Prep and drape the skin.
4. Insert finder needle and syringe, at 30–45° angle, constantly pulling back on the plunger. Aim towards the ipsilateral nipple.
   (a) Aiming laterally avoids puncturing the carotid artery.
   (b) If you hit the carotid artery, pull the needle out completely and apply pressure for 3–5 min.
5. Fan the needle in and out slowly until dark blood is drawn back easily in the syringe.
6. Carefully switch hands to hold the finder needle and syringe with the left hand. Rest the left hand against the patient to minimize movement.
7. Now pick up the introducer needle and syringe with your right hand.
8. Insert the introducer needle and syringe into the skin at 1 o'clock relative to the finder needle, following the same 30–45° angle and aiming towards the ipsilateral needle.
9. Draw back on plunger and advance needle until have return of dark blood.
10. Switch hands to hold the introducer needle and syringe with the left hand.
11. Remove the finder needle and syringe completely.
12. Gently disconnect the introducer syringe from the introducer needle using your right hand. Continue to hold the introducer needle in place with your left hand.
13. Ensure no pulsatile flow.
14. Smoothly thread guidewire through the introducer needle.

15. Remove introducer needle over the guidewire.
16. Advance manometry catheter over the guidewire.
17. Remove guidewire from the manometry catheter.
18. Gently connect manometry tubing to manometry catheter.
19. Hold the manometry tubing down to allow it to fill by gravity.
20. Once full, then elevate the tubing up. Should NOT see the tubing continue to fill up.
    (a) The height of the column is pressure in cmH_2O. Divide this height by 1.36 to convert to mmHg.*
21. Disconnect the manometry tubing.
22. Thread the guidewire through the manometry catheter.
23. Remove the manometry catheter.
24. Make a skin nick with the scalpel.
25. Advance the central line catheter (e.g., Cordis, double, or triple lumen) over the guidewire, in a twisting motion.
26. Remove the guidewire.
27. Attach flushes and ensure all ports draw back blood and flush easily.
28. Attach luer lock caps or stopcocks.
29. Secure central line with suture.
30. Secure with biopatch, tegaderm.

*Conversion factor: Mercury (Hg) is 13.6 times the density of water (H_2O), and 10 mm = 1 cm. To convert cmH_2O to mmHg, divide by 1.36.

Femoral Lines Without Ultrasound **25**

Indications for Femoral Central Line Placement

1. Least sterile, less ideal traditionally compared to subclavian and internal jugular central lines
2. Subclavian central line contraindications: broken clavicle, difficulty placing due to anatomy, body habitus
3. Internal jugular central line contraindications: cervical collar, elevated ICP/neurosurgical case
4. No access to neck/chest: intraoperative placement during ENT or neurosurgical case, active chest compressions during CPR

Indications for Femoral Arterial Line Placement

1. Unable to place arterial line in smaller artery like radial, brachial, or pedal artery
2. Anticipated loss of smaller peripheral arterial line
   (a) Vasoplegia
   (b) Circulatory arrest during cardiopulmonary bypass

Patient Positioning

- Supine with legs extended or frogleg position with hip abducted can be helpful; roll under posterior superior iliac crests can help with approach by extending hip.
- Flat.
- If obese body habitus, tape the pannus upward to expose the inguinal crease and create flat surface. Skin folds will interfere with identifying landmarks.

© The Author(s), under exclusive license to Springer Nature Switzerland AG 2021   123
C. Sampankanpanich Soria et al., *Anesthesiology Resident Manual of Procedures*,
https://doi.org/10.1007/978-3-030-65732-1_25

Femoral Arterial Line

1. Equipment: Femoral arterial line kit
   (a) Introducer needle
   (b) +/− Syringe
   (c) Guidewire
   (d) Catheter
   (e) Suture
   (f) Scalpel
   (g) Biopatch
   (h) Tegaderm
   (i) Sterile gauze
   (j) Sterile gloves
   (k) Large chloraprep stick
   (l) Sterile flush and pigtail tubing
2. Identify landmarks: inguinal crease, pubic symphysis, and anterior superior iliac spine.
3. Draw an imaginary line between the ASIS and pubic symphysis.
4. Insertion site is below the inguinal crease, midway between the ASIS and pubic symphysis.
5. Using left index and middle fingers, palpate the femoral pulse.
6. Imagine the neurovascular bundle:
   (a) Lateral-N-A-V-E-L-Medial "NAVEL toward the navel"
   (b) Lateral-Nerve-Artery-Vein-Empty-Lymphatics-Medial
7. Insertion site: where the pulse is felt.
8. Angle:
   (a) Using your right hand, insert the introducer needle with or without the syringe at 30° angle.
   (b) Aim toward the path of the artery, toward the umbilicus.
   (c) Aim steeper if larger patient with more subcutaneous tissue.
9. Fan the needle in and out slowly until bright red blood, pulsatile flow is seen.
   (a) If hit vein, pull needle back to skin and aim more laterally. Small adjustments.
   (b) If using needle alone, advance until seeing pulsatile flow through the needle. If it's a dribble, the needle bevel is not entirely in the femoral artery lumen.
   (c) If using needle with syringe attached, constantly pull back on the plunger until bright red blood is seen filling up the syringe easily.
10. Carefully switch to holding the needle with your left hand. Brace your left hand against the patient to ensure stability.
11. Using your right hand, advance the guidewire through the needle. Should pass easily without resistance.
12. Remove the needle over the guidewire.
13. +/− Make a small skin nick with the scalpel.
14. Advance the catheter over the guidewire.
15. Secure with suture, biopatch, and tegaderm.

Femoral Central Line

1. Equipment: central line kit
   (a) Introducer needle and syringe
   (b) Guidewire
   (c) Manometry catheter and tubing
   (d) Catheter (e.g., Cordis, double lumen, triple lumen)
   (e) Scalpel
   (f) Suture
   (g) Biopatch
   (h) Tegaderm
   (i) Sterile gauze
   (j) Sterile flushes
   (k) Caps for catheter (e.g. luer lock caps, stopcocks)
2. Identify landmarks: inguinal crease, pubic symphysis, and anterior superior iliac spine.
3. Draw an imaginary line between the ASIS and pubic symphysis.
4. Insertion site is below the inguinal crease, midway between the ASIS and pubic symphysis.
5. Using left index and middle fingers, palpate the femoral pulse.
6. Imagine the neurovascular bundle:
   (a) Lateral-N-A-V-E-L-Medial
   (b) Lateral-Nerve-Artery-Vein-Empty-Lymphatics-Medial
7. Insertion site: 1–1.5 cm medial to where the pulse is felt
8. Angle:
   (a) Insert the introducer needle and syringe at 30° angle, constantly pulling back on the plunger.
   (b) Aim toward the path of the blood vessel, toward the umbilicus.
   (c) Aim steeper if larger patient with more subcutaneous tissue.
9. Fan the needle in and out slowly until dark blood is drawn back easily in the syringe.
10. Gently disconnect the syringe from the introducer needle.
11. Ensure no pulsatile flow.
12. Smoothly thread guidewire through the introducer needle.
13. Remove introducer needle over the guidewire.
14. Advance manometry catheter over the guidewire.
15. Remove guidewire from the manometry catheter.
16. Gently connect manometry tubing to manometry catheter.
17. Hold the manometry tubing down to allow it to fill by gravity.
18. Once full, then elevate the tubing up. Should NOT see the tubing continue to fill up.
    (a) The height of the column is pressure in cmH_2O. Divide this height by 1.36 to convert to mmHg.*
19. Disconnect the manometry tubing.
20. Thread the guidewire through the manometry catheter.
21. Remove the manometry catheter.

22. Make a skin nick with the scalpel.
23. Advance the central line catheter (e.g., Cordis, double or triple lumen) over the guidewire in a twisting motion.
24. Remove the guidewire.
25. Attach flushes and ensure that all ports draw back blood and flush easily.
26. Attach luer lock caps or stopcocks.
27. Secure central line with suture.
28. Secure with biopatch, tegaderm.

*Conversion factor: Mercury (Hg) is 13.6 times the density of water (H_2O) and 10 mm = 1 cm. To convert cmH_2O to mmHg, divide by 1.36.

How to Assemble an Arterial Line Transducer

26

Equipment

1. Pressure bag
2. 500 cc bag of normal saline
3. Pressure tubing +/− vamp
4. Pressure transducer cable and monitor

Instructions

1. Compress the vamp and evacuate all air (Fig. 26.3).
2. Spike the 500 cc bag of normal saline with the pressure tubing (Fig. 26.1)/(Fig. 26.2)/(Fig. 26.4).
3. Fill up the tubing chamber with normal saline by squeezing the chamber.
4. Place the normal saline bag in the pressure bag.
5. Pull the tab on the pressure tubing to fill up the tubing with saline completely. Ensure all air bubbles are flushed through.
6. Inflate the pressure bag until the green line shows (Fig. 26.5).
7. Connect the pressure tubing to the transducer cable.
8. Turn on monitor.
9. Open the cap on the transducer stopcock.
10. Close the stopcock to the patient.
11. Click "Zero ABP" or "Zero ART" on the monitor.
12. When zeroing is completed, put the cap back on the stopcock and close the stopcock to the cap.
13. Ready for use.

© The Author(s), under exclusive license to Springer Nature Switzerland AG 2021
C. Sampankanpanich Soria et al., *Anesthesiology Resident Manual of Procedures*,
https://doi.org/10.1007/978-3-030-65732-1_26

Fig. 26.1 Photograph of
primed arterial line
pressure tubing

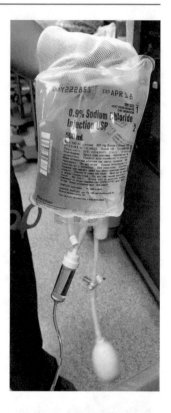

Fig. 26.2 Demonstration
of how to flush pressure
line tubing by pulling the
blue tab at the transducer

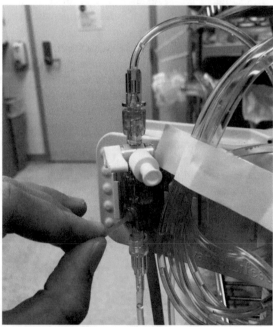

Fig. 26.3 Prior to flushing the tubing, close the vamp completely so that there are no air bubbles

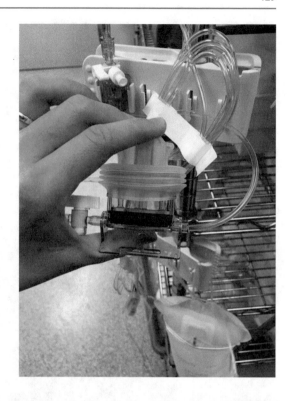

Fig. 26.4 Make sure the chamber is completely full, with no air

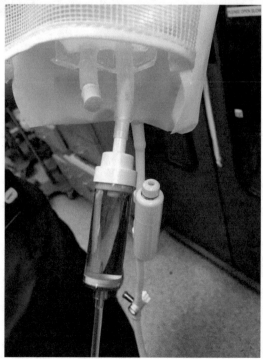

Fig. 26.5 Pressurize the
bag until the green
line shows

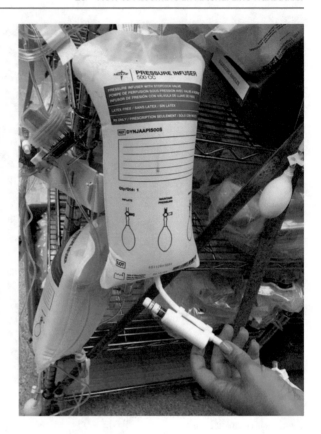

Radial Arterial Lines

27

Indications

- Consistent and continuous monitoring of BP
- Hemodynamically unstable
- Titration of inotropic and vasopressor medications
- Frequent blood sampling
- Frequent arterial blood gases
- Significant ventilator deficits

Contraindications

- Should not compromise circulation distal to placement site
- Avoid sites with known deficiencies in collateral circulation (e.g. Raynaud's, thromboangitis, end arteries)
- Allen's test: verifies collateral circulation via radial and ulnar arteries: controversial utility
- Infection at intended site of catheter placement
- Traumatic injury proximal to site of insertion

Equipment for Self-Assembled Radial Arterial Line Kit

1. Sterile gloves
2. Blue towels
3. Saline flush and pigtail tubing with stopcock
4. Arm board
5. Roll: rolled gauze, rolled blue towel, tape roll, foam cushion
6. Sterile gauze
7. Small chloraprep

© The Author(s), under exclusive license to Springer Nature Switzerland AG 2021
C. Sampankanpanich Soria et al., *Anesthesiology Resident Manual of Procedures*,
https://doi.org/10.1007/978-3-030-65732-1_27

8. Tape
9. Tegaderm
10. Bipoatch
11. 1% lidocaine on TB syringe needle in case of awake patient
12. 20 G angiocath or Arrow needles (personal preference)
13. Guidewire (personal preference)
14. Tray table or mayo stand
15. Arterial line transducer setup

Instructions

1. Palpate radial pulses on both arms.
2. Assuming no contraindications to placement, start with the arm with the strongest palpable pulse.
3. If the BP cuff is on the same side, switch the BP cuff to the opposite arm so that you still have NIBP readings. Otherwise, cycle the cuff less frequently.
4. Place the arm board and roll around the patient's posterior forearm (Fig. 27.1)/(Fig 27.2).
   (a) The roll should be positioned underneath the distal wrist, putting the wrist in extension.
   (b) Place the distal strap of the armboard across the thenar eminence, extending the thumb.
   (c) Be careful not to extend the wrist too much, as this will compress the radial artery, decreasing the lumen size and decreasing pulsatile flow.

Fig. 27.1 (a/b) Position the forearm and wrist on an armboard with a roll underneath the wrist for extension and a strap across the thumb

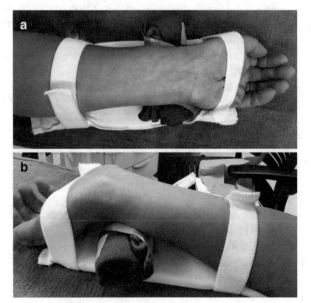

Fig. 27.2 (**a/b**) If an armboard and roll are not available, the foam cushion for the usual OR table armboard can be folded over and taped

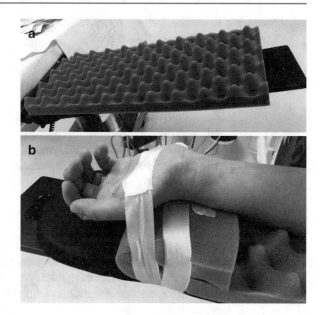

5. Clean the skin with chloraprep.
6. Awake patient: topicalize generously with 1% lidocaine. Use non-sterile gloves.
    (a) Arterial lines are painful due to the innervations around the radial artery.
    (b) Draw up 1 cc or 3 cc syringe of 1% lidocaine and attach to TB syringe needle.
    (c) At the intended site of needle placement, inject lidocaine to create a generous skin wheal.
    (d) Keeping the needle in the same site, slowly draw back the needle tip to the skin. Angle the needle to the right of the artery and inject another skin wheal.
    (e) Draw the needle tip back again to the skin, and angle to the left of the artery, and inject another skin wheal.
7. Clean the skin again with chloraprep.
8. Put on sterile gloves.
9. Drape the area with blue towels to expand sterile field.
10. Take out guidewire from packaging and have it available close by.
11. Palpate the pulse with the tips of the left index and middle fingers.
    (a) Use as small a surface area as possible to better pinpoint the location of the radial artery.
12. Hold the catheter/needle in the right hand like a pencil at a 30–45° angle.
    (a) The steeper the angle, the smaller the surface area of bevel exposed to arterial flow, and the harder it is to thread the guidewire.
13. Advance in and out slowly until flash of blood is seen in the catheter.
    (a) If no flash is seen, draw needle tip to the skin, and angle slightly medial or lateral in the direction of the pulse.
    (b) Continue to advance in and out until flash is obtained.
    (c) Small movements, especially in a patient with a small radial artery.

14. Once flash is obtained, decide whether to follow through-and-through technique or direct catheter advancement.
    (a) Through-and-through
        (i) Pros: easy to do, works well for small flash or large flash.
        (ii) Cons: risk hematoma, must be done quickly.
        (iii) Technique:
            1. Once flash is obtained, keep the needle in the same trajectory and advance deeper until flash disappears.
            2. Hold the catheter with the left hand.
            3. Use the right hand to remove the needle.
            4. With the right hand, pick up the guidewire and position close to the catheter, ready for insertion.
            5. With the left hand, slowly and carefully remove the catheter until pulsatile flow of blood is seen coming through the catheter.
            6. With the right hand, thread the guidewire slowly through the catheter. The guidewire should advance easily with no resistance.
            7. Thread the catheter over the guidewire. It should advance smoothly with no resistance. A gentle twisting motion helps the catheter advance through skin.
    (b) Arrow catheter
        (i) Pros: guidewire built into the catheter, less hematoma, less mess/blood loss
        (ii) Cons: institutional availability, takes practice
        (iii) Technique:
            1. Once flash is obtained, flatten the needle and advance 1 mm in a slight twisting/screw motion.
            2. Verify that blood is still filling up in the catheter.
            3. Slowly slide the guidewire into the artery by advancing the black cap.
            4. Advance the catheter over the guidewire and into the artery in a slight twisting motion.
            5. Pull the guidewire and needle out of the catheter.
            6. Everything should advance smoothly.
    (c) Direct catheter advancement
        (i) Pros: don't need Arrow catheter, if fails can revert to through-and-through technique, less hematoma, less mess/blood loss
        (ii) Cons: takes practice, need good flow
        (iii) Technique:
            1. Once flash is obtained, flatten the needle and advance 1 mm in a slight twisting motion.
            2. Verify that blood is still filling up in the catheter.
            3. Slowly slide the catheter into the artery lumen. Use a twisting motion to help advance through the skin.
            4. Everything should advance smoothly.
            5. Remove the needle.

15. Hold pressure on the artery to minimize blood loss.
    (a) Apply pressure with three fingers over the forearm:
        (i) Index finger at insertion site
        (ii) Middle finger at distal end of catheter (visualize where it terminates in the forearm)
        (iii) Ring finger proximal to catheter
    (b) Use the palm of the left hand to push on the forearm proximally.
16. Attach pigtail and sterile flush to catheter. Ensure tight connections.
    (a) Warm room: plastic expands, a loose connection still feels tight.
    (b) Cold operating room: plastic shrinks, a loose connection is now loose, leaks under the drapes, bad arterial waveform, and unintended blood loss.
    (c) Pull back on the syringe: bright red blood should draw back easily and fill the syringe.
    (d) Flush the syringe: artery should flush easily without resistance.
17. Secure arterial line with biopatch, tegaderm, and tape.
18. Connect to transducer.

Troubleshooting Radial Arterial Lines

1. Be patient. Arterial lines are humbling.
2. Resistance advancing the guidewire
    (a) Not entirely in the lumen, but at the sidewall. May need to attempt a new insertion site.
    (b) Not truly pulsatile flow. Remove the guidewire and pull back on the catheter a little more until pulsatile flow is obtained.
    (c) Calcification, atherosclerosis of the radial artery. Visible under ultrasound. Common in elderly, comorbid conditions like coronary artery disease and end-stage renal disease, smokers. May need a smaller guidewire or try a more proximal insertion site.
    (d) Artery curves. Likely inserted too distal where the artery is more superficial, stronger pulse, but there's a curvature. May need to try a more proximal insertion site.
    (e) Artery may be in vasospasm from multiple attempts. Try a more proximal insertion site or go to the other arm.
3. Pulsatile flow and guidewire advances easily, but resistance advancing catheter over the guidewire.
    (a) Try a gentle twisting motion. Patient may have thick skin. Caution: do not force. May dissect the artery.
4. Small tiny flash.
    (a) Patient may have small radial artery or poor flow.
    (b) If there's a flash, always try it out. Small flash can still mean the catheter is in the artery lumen.
    (c) To improve flash visualization, flush the needle with saline. A small drop of blood will appear more dramatically.

5. No flash despite advancing in and out at different angles.
    (a) Needle may be clotted by blood, fat, skin debris from multiple advancements.
    (b) Remove the needle completely and flush with saline.
6. Dampened waveform.
    (a) Dislodged arterial line.
    (b) Clotted arterial line. Try power flush with 0.5–1 cc of normal saline.
7. Unable to feel a pulse, or a very weak pulse.
    (a) Low threshold to use ultrasound, especially in certain patient populations (end-stage renal disease, anticoagulated status, etc.).

When to Check an Arterial Blood Gas

1. After interventions
    (a) Changing ventilator settings
    (b) Transfusing blood products
    (c) Treatment of metabolic abnormalities
2. Depends on patient and type/duration of procedure
    (a) Q1hr is a general good rule of thumb
3. If suspect changes
    (a) Major blood lass
    (b) Electrolyte derangements
    (b) Acid-base disturbances
4. If diabetic, check glucose q1hr

Utility of Venous Blood Gas

1. Reasonable approximation of $PaCO_2$, pH and base access.
2. Saves an arterial puncture.
3. Venous PCO_2 is ~4–6 mmHg higher than arterial PCO_2.
4. Venous pH is ~0.03–0.04 lower than arterial pH.
5. Cannot be used to estimate oxygenation because venous PO_2 is significantly lower than PO_2 and varies depending on site of venous blood draw and level of metabolic activity.
6. Faster results than ABG: good for assessment of Hb/Hct.

Dorsal Pedal Arterial Lines

28

Pedal Versus Radial Arterial Lines

1. Intraoperative placement and unable to access arms because tucked or under drapes.
2. Unable to place radial arterial line (clot, vasospasm, prior attempts unsuccessful).
3. Desire to avoid cannulating femoral artery.

Equipment for Self-Assembled Pedal Arterial Line Kit

1. Sterile gloves
2. Blue towels
3. Saline flush and pigtail tubing with stopcock
4. Sterile gauze
5. Small chloraprep
6. Tape
7. Tegaderm
8. Bipoatch
9. 1% lidocaine on TB syringe needle in case of awake patient
10. 20 G angiocath or Arrow needles (personal preference)
11. Guidewire (personal preference)
12. Tray table or mayo stand
13. Arterial line transducer setup

C. Sampankanpanich Soria et al., *Anesthesiology Resident Manual of Procedures*,
https://doi.org/10.1007/978-3-030-65732-1_28

Instructions

1. Palpate dorsal pedal pulses on both feet.
2. Assuming no contraindications to placement, start with the foot with the strongest palpable pulse. This is an end artery, but when other options not available, it is often used.
3. Tape the foot down across the big toe to hold the foot in position. Do not tape too tightly as this will flatten the artery.
4. Clean the skin with chloraprep.
5. Put on sterile gloves.
6. Drape the area with blue towels to expand sterile field.
7. Take out guidewire from packaging and have it available close by.
8. Palpate the pulse with the tips of the left index and middle fingers.
    (a) Use as small a surface area as possible to better pinpoint the location of the radial artery.
9. Hold the catheter/needle in the right hand like a pencil at a 30° angle.
    (a) Key to pedal arterial lines is to stay as flat as possible.
    (b) Ensure the insertion site provides enough room to angle the needle.
    (c) If you start too distal, the artery will curve and your hand will hit the patient's toes.
    (d) If you start too proximal, you have a stronger pulse but shorter territory for error.
10. Advance in and out slowly until flash of blood is seen in the catheter.
    (a) If no flash is seen, draw needle tip to the skin and angle slightly medial or lateral in the direction of the pulse.
    (b) Continue to advance in and out until flash is obtained.
11. Once flash is obtained, the through-and-through technique is the easiest method.
    (a) The hardest part is having a long and straight enough artery to advance the guidewire.
    (b) Once flash is obtained, keep the needle in the same trajectory and advance deeper until flash disappears.
    (c) Hold the catheter with the left hand.
    (d) Use the right hand to remove the needle.
    (e) With the right hand, pick up the guidewire and position close to the catheter, ready for insertion.
    (f) With the left hand, slowly and carefully remove the catheter until pulsatile flow of blood is seen coming through the catheter.
    (g) With the right hand, thread the guidewire slowly through the catheter. The guidewire should advance easily with no resistance.
    (h) Thread the catheter over the guidewire. It should advance smoothly with no resistance. A gentle twisting motion helps the catheter advance through skin.

12. Hold pressure on the artery to minimize blood loss.
    (a) Apply pressure with three fingers over the forearm:
        (i) Index finger at insertion site
        (ii) Middle finger at distal end of catheter (visualize where it terminates in the forearm)
        (iii) Ring finger proximal to catheter
    (b) Use the palm of the left hand to push on the foot proximally.
13. Attach pigtail and sterile flush to catheter. Ensure tight connections.
    (a) Warm room: plastic expands, a loose connection still feels tight.
    (b) Cold operating room: plastic shrinks, a loose connection is now loose, leaks under the drapes, bad arterial waveform, and unintended blood loss.
    (c) Pull back on the syringe: bright red blood should draw back easily and fill the syringe.
    (d) Flush the syringe: artery should flush easily without resistance.
14. Secure arterial line with Biopatch® and Tegaderm®, and tape.
15. Connect to transducer.

Belmont Infuser

29

What Is the Belmont?

- Rapid Infuser RI-2 is a rapid infusion system for use in high blood loss surgical procedures, trauma, and any situation where rapid replacement and warming of blood or fluids is required (Fig. 29.1).
- Standard practice is to use the larger 3.0 L reservoir to maximize infusion volumes.
- Quick and easy to set up. Instructions appear on the screen when first turned on. Only takes 13 s to prime system tubing, ideally using 200 cc of normal saline.
- Dual patient line to maximize infusion rates.
- Roller-type peristaltic pump to prevent blood clots.

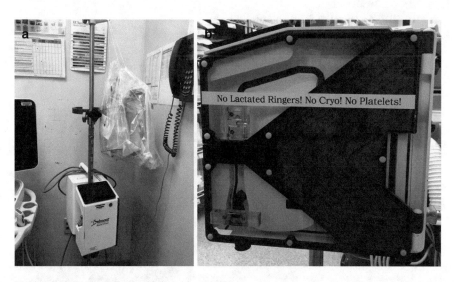

Fig. 29.1 (**a/b**) Photograph of a Belmont machine

© The Author(s), under exclusive license to Springer Nature Switzerland AG 2021   141
C. Sampankanpanich Soria et al., *Anesthesiology Resident Manual of Procedures*,
https://doi.org/10.1007/978-3-030-65732-1_29

How Does the Belmont Stop Air and Blood Clots?

- Two air detectors: air is automatically detected, removed, and released into the room air
- Pressure sensor
  - Continuously displays
  - Stops infusion at >300 mmHg OR sudden pressure spike
  - Slows flow rate to safe line pressure
- Two temperature probes (prevent cold, prevent clots)
- Pump infusion rate sensor
- Open door detector
- Valve activation sensors
- Recirculation
  - Automatically recirculates blood while actively infusing and while in standby mode
  - Only stops if Belmont machine is powered off
  - Option to press "RECIRC" button to manually recirculate blood at rate of 200 ml/min

How to Set Up the Belmont

1. Plug in the Belmont machine and turn on the power switch. Follow step by step instructions on the screen (Fig. 29.2).
2. Gather tubing and reservoir kit (Fig. 29.3).
   (a) 3 L reservoir
   (b) Tubing to spike fluid and blood bags
   (c) Tubing to pass through Belmont machine
3. Set reservoir into the holder.
   (a) Most providers switch to the larger 3 L reservoir in order to transfuse larger fluid volumes.

Fig. 29.2 Photograph of the start-up screen when a Belmont machine is first turned on

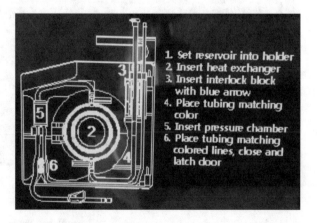

1. Set reservoir into holder
2. Insert heat exchanger
3. Insert interlock block with blue arrow
4. Place tubing matching color
5. Insert pressure chamber
6. Place tubing matching colored lines, close and latch door

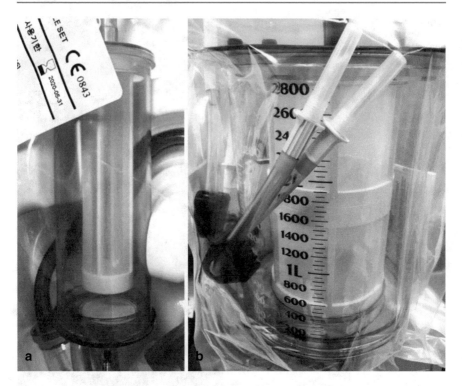

Fig. 29.3 (**a/b**) Photographs of small and large 3-L reservoirs for the Belmont machine

4. Connect spiking tubing to top of reservoir (Fig. 29.4).
   (a) Total of five ports.
   (b) Remove blue cap, push spiking tubing onto the port tightly and securely.
   (c) Tape the spiking tubing cap to the top of the reservoir, so don't lose caps.
   (d) Clamp the spiking tubing closed when not in use.
5. Connect pressure tubing to tail on bottom reservoir (Fig. 29.5).
   (a) Make sure this connection screws together tightly.
6. Insert the pressure tubing into the Belmont box (Fig. 29.6).
   (a) Everything is color-coded with arrows.
7. Connect pressure to double extension tubing going to patient.
8. Prime tubing with minimum 200 cc of fluid to prevent air entrainment.
   (a) Spike a 1 L bag of normal saline.
   (b) Do NOT use lactated ringers.
   (c) Leave the 1 L bag of NS hanging.
9. Program infusion rate based on catheter size.
   (a) 20 G – 100 ml/min
   (b) 18 G – 200 ml/min
   (c) 16 G – 400 ml/min
   (d) 14 G – 750 ml/min
   (e) 12 G – 1000 ml/min

Fig. 29.4 Photograph of
IV tubing spiked and
connected to the reservoir
chamber of a
Belmont machine

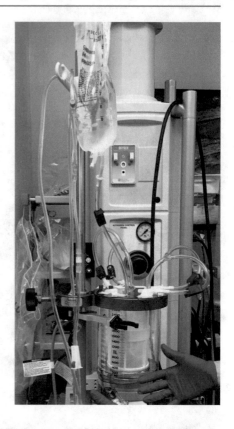

Fig. 29.5 Photograph of
pressure tubing connecting
bottom of reservoir to the
Belmont box

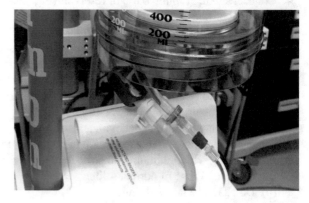

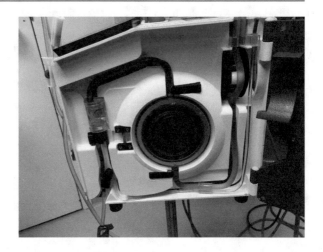

Fig. 29.6 Photograph of pressure tubing inserted into the Belmont box

10. Connect to patient.
11. Begin infusing products.
    (a) Do NOT use cryoprecipitate.
    (b) Do NOT use platelets.

Causes of High-Pressure Alarm

1. Patient line is occluded.
2. Recirculation line is blocked.
3. Infusion site is not well placed.

Management: inspect the patient and recirculation lines to make sure that the flow path is not blocked.

Single Shot Spinal

30

The following tables outline approaches to placing a spinal (Table 30.1), dosing a spinal (Table 30.2), common complications of spinal blocks (Table 30.3), and assessment of level of neuraxial blockade (Table 30.4).

Placing a Spinal

Dosing a Spinal

Complications of Spinal Block

Assessing Block Level

© The Author(s), under exclusive license to Springer Nature Switzerland AG 2021
C. Sampankanpanich Soria et al., *Anesthesiology Resident Manual of Procedures*,
https://doi.org/10.1007/978-3-030-65732-1_30

Table 30.1 Instructions for positioning a patient properly for spinal placement

Position of patient	Sitting	Ideal position is sitting. Contraindicated if patient too sick, unstable, physically unable to sit. Manually sit if anatomy is too difficult supine. Two extra providers push up on patient's back and shoulder while you place spinal block.	Lateral supine	More comfortable to patient. Challenges: obese, pregnant, large hips → curves spinal column. May require paramedian approach if midline too difficult.
Needle type	Pencil point	Messier cut, dura heals faster, lower risk of post-dural puncture headache (PDPH). Not sharp enough to cut skin by itself; requires introducer needle first; slower technique.	Quincke, cutting	Sharper cut, dura doesn't heal as quickly, so higher risk of Post-dural puncture headache (PDPH). Cuts skin by itself; don't need introducer needle; faster technique.
Approach to insertion	Midline	Identify correct space. Use marking pen to help orient yourself. Go between spinous processes. Flatter angle, parallel to ground in lumbar region. More cephalad, steeper angle in thoracic region.	Paramedian	Identify correct space. Use marking pen to help orient yourself. Insert 1–1.5 cm off midline to right or left of interspace. Aim straight, parallel to ground. Goal is to hit lamina, then advance in and out, toward midline and cephalad, until hit spinous process, then cephalad through interspinous ligament, then ligamentum flavum, then intrathecal space. Faster to use Quincke needle

Table 30.2 Instructions for dosing a spinal based on baricity of local anesthetic, type of local anesthetic, and combination with opioids

Baricity	Isobaric	Cannot adjust dermatome level by repositioning patient. Local anesthetic solution stays where it was injected. Longer duration of action than hyperbaric.
	Hyperbaric	Contains dextrose (5–8%) For more cephalad spread, may carefully tilt patient in slight Trendelenburg position if needed to follow natural lordosis of thoracic spine. HOWEVER, be sure to elevate head and cervical spine to avoid high spinal.
	Hypobaric	Infrequently used. Prone patient, inject solution, rises to top. Can adjust dermatome level by repositioning patient.

Table 30.2 (continued)

Patient positioning	Only works for hyperbaric and hypobaric solutions.	
Local anesthetic	Lidocaine	More motor block than bupivacaine. Not used as often as in the past due to lidocaine neurotoxicity and risk of transient neurologic syndrome especially with higher concentrations of lidocaine injecate
	Bupivacaine	Most commonly used Potency of block depends on dose used. Kit vial: 2 cc of 0.75% hyperbaric bupivacaine
Opioid	Fentanyl	Commonly used intrathecal narcotic. Prolongs block duration. Risks: respiratory depression, nausea, vomiting, pruritus, urinary retention.

Table 30.3 Common complications of a spinal block, including risk factors, etiology, and timeline of development

Sympathetic blockade	Sympathetic fibers: T1 to L2. Beta cardiac-accelerator fibers: left side T1 to T5. Level of block: sympathetic > sensory > motor. Aka: autonomics > pain, temperature > touch, proprioception > motor. Hypotension primarily from decreased venous preload, less so from arterial vasodilation. Alpha blockers → vasodilate veins and arteries. Extreme caution/contraindications: severe aortic stenosis. Sudden, dramatic loss of preload → systemic hypotension → decreased coronary perfusion pressure → decreased cardiac output. Bradycardia is a real phenomenon. Sometimes ignored/denied by provider. Prevention: ondansetron 8 mg IV prior to intrathecal injection. Co-load vs. pre-load with crystalloids to prevent hypotension.
Post-dural puncture headache	Approximately 1% incidence with 25G pencil-point spinal needle. Pressure gradient and opening from dural puncture → CSF leak, pulling on meninges, and compensatory cerebral vasodilation. Risk factors: young, thin, Quincke cutting needle
Transient neurologic symptoms	Associated with lidocaine when used intrathecally. Symptoms: pain in lower back, buttocks, lower extremities; no motor deficits. Timeline: develops within 6 h post-spinal, generally resolves spontaneously within days to months. Risk factors: outpatient procedures, lithotomy position.
Hematoma	Risk factors: traumatic placement, coagulation status of patient (warfarin, ESLD, etc.) Fear: progression to cauda equine syndrome = surgical emergency. New onset radicular back pain, saddle anesthetic, bowel/bladder incontinence, lower extremity weakness.

Table 30.4 Techniques for evaluating level of sensory blockade

Stimulus	Cold	Glove of ice	Sharp	Broken tongue depressor
		Alcohol prep stick		Nail cleaner from scrub sponge
Change in stimulus	Report a change	Start low and work up. "Tell me when it starts to feel sharp/cold."	This or that	"Cold or pressure?" "Sharp or pressure?" Side to side comparison in case asymmetric coverage.

Lumbar Epidurals

31

Spinal Cord Anatomy

1. Spinal cord terminates at L1 (on average): from foramen magnum to filum terminale.
2. Iliac crest corresponds to L4 vertebral body or L4–L5 interspace.
3. Blood supply
   (a) 1 anterior spinal artery +2 posterior spinal arteries = longitudinal pathways
       (i) Anterior spinal artery arises from vertebral artery caudal to basilar artery. ASA supplies 75% of blood supply to spinal cord. It is much more vulnerable than posterior spinal arteries.
   (b) Segmental arteries of the vertebral column supply radicular arteries
       (i) Aorta
       (ii) Costocervical and intercostal arteries in thorax
       (iii) Lumbar and iliolumbar arteries in lumbar region
       (iv) Lateral sacral arteries in pelvis
       (v) Artery of Adamkiewicz: largest segmental artery; located in lower thoracic–upper lumbar region, position varies from T7 to L4; usually T10 on left side

Dermatome Coverage

- Early labor: visceral, T10 to L2
- Spontaneous vaginal delivery including an episiotomy: somatic, S2–S4
- Forceps-assisted vaginal delivery: T10 to S4 (tugging on uterus on ovaries)
- Cesarean section: up to T4
  - Beginning, cut uterus and remove baby: up to T10
  - After baby is out, evert uterus: up to T4
- Postpartum tubal ligation: up to T4

© The Author(s), under exclusive license to Springer Nature Switzerland AG 2021
C. Sampankanpanich Soria et al., *Anesthesiology Resident Manual of Procedures*,
https://doi.org/10.1007/978-3-030-65732-1_31

Key Dermatome Landmarks to Know

- Umbilicus: T10
- Xiphoid process: T6
- Nipples: T4
- Armpit: T2
- Shoulder tip: C4
- Back of knee: S2

Patient Positioning

1. Supine, right or left lateral decubitus
   (a) Curl patient as much as possible, bringing knees and chin to chest, to open up lumbar space as much as possible
   (b) Indications: patient unable to sit
      (i) Active labor, pushing
2. Sitting
   (a) Ideal, most common and easiest positioning for provider
   (b) What to tell patient:
      (i) Arms crossed in lap, can hug a pillow for comfort.
      (ii) Slouch forward, like bad posture.
      (iii) Round out the lower back, push the provider's hand away at lower back.
   (c) Double check that patient is truly flat. OB beds are lumpy and downsloping, meant to be broken down into stirrups for vaginal delivery. Use blankets under hips to make patient even.
   (d) If struggling to find interspace, reassess patient positioning.
      (i) Is patient scared, leaning forward away from the needle?
      (ii) Is patient in pain, rocking around?

Insertion and Depth

1. Palpate iliac crests = L4–L5 interspace or L4 vertebral body.
2. Choosing an interspace:
   (a) L3–L4 interspace is usually easier, wider.
   (b) L4–L5 interspace is usually tighter, harder to get to with Touhy needle and smaller space to thread epidural catheter. Benefit is better coverage of sacral area.
3. Goal is for Touhy to be fixed in ligament. No point advancing Touhy needle and injecting saline into subcutaneous tissue.
4. If obese patients, may be difficult to palpate bony structures.
   (a) Use local as a finder needle, try to hit spinous process to find midline.
   (b) Look at C7 cervical prominence in neck and sacrum. Draw a line between the two. That is roughly midline.

(c) Subcutaneous tissue may fall to the sides laterally. Center is midline.
5. Always try to estimate the depth of loss of resistance (LOR).
   (a) Thin patient, may be as shallow as 3.5 cm.
   (b) Obese patient, may be as deep as 7 cm.
   (c) General rule of thumb: insert Touhy with stylette to 3 cm, then remove Stylette and use LOR syringe.
6. Do not inject too much saline as you advance Touhy needle. Will run out of saline in the epidural kit and make it difficult to palpate landmarks.
7. Hitting bone:
   (a) Hitting bone early is usually spinous process. Angle up or down, depending whether you're too low or too high in the interspace.
   (b) Hitting bone late is usually lamina. Angle cephalad and left or right toward midline.
8. Small angles outside = big angles inside.

Loss of Resistance (LOR) Techniques

I. Intermittent Pressure and Advancement
   (a) Fill syringe with saline and air
   (b) Advance – Check LOR – Advance – Check LOR
   (c) Check LOR by bouncing on the syringe
   (d) Advance 1–2 mm at a time with Touhy needle
   (e) Keep alternating until have LOR, then thread epidural catheter
   (f) How deep to leave catheter at skin: distance to LOR + 3–5 cm
II. Continuous Pressure
   (a) Push on the syringe with your right thumb, holding constant pressure, while simultaneously advancing the Touhy needle with your left hand, until encountering LOR.
   (b) Caution: must apply equal pressure on syringe and Touhy needle, otherwise will advance Touhy needle too fast and enter intrathecal space.

Lumbar Epidural for Labor

1. Loading dose:
   (a) Medication:
       (i) Drug: 0.125% or 0.25% bupivacaine ± 50 mcg fentanyl.
       (ii) Volume: 8–10 cc depending on patient height.
   (b) Always cycle blood pressure cuff.
   (c) Remain in the room or check back on patient frequently.
2. Bad things that happen with epidural loading:
   (a) Remember: uterine perfusion pressure = mean arterial pressure minus uterine pressure.

(b) Sympathetic block from local anesthetic → vasodilation → maternal hypotension → decrease in uterine perfusion pressure → fetal heart rate deceleration.

(c) Sympathetic block → lack of pain stimulus → maternal hypotension + sleepy mom → decrease in uterine perfusion pressure → fetal heart rate deceleration.

(d) Sympathetic block → lack of epinephrine and norepinephrine → lack of beta-2 agonist effects → uterine muscle contraction → increased uterine pressure → decreased uterine perfusion pressure → fetal heart rate deceleration. If uterine tetany is suspected cause of fetal distress, immediately administer 400–800 mcg sublingual nitroglycerine spray.

Lumbar Epidural for Cesarean Section

1. Anesthetic considerations for prolonged labor, now going for cesarean section (Fig. 31.1).
   - Higher risk of uterine atony and postpartum hemorrhage
   - Higher risk of chorioamnionitis and sepsis → hypotension, tachycardia, fever, uterine atony

Epidural Options for Cesarean

- Extend T10 level of *analgesia* to T4 level of *anesthesia*

- Usually requires 10-20 ml volume w/ adjuvants

  - Depending on pre-existing sensory level and block density

- 20 cc of chlorprocaine 3% w/ bicarb

  - Works fast b/c large dose

  - Resolves quickly b/c breakdown by pseudocholinesterase

  - Must redose within 20 min

- 2% lidocaine w/ bicarb common for non-emergent

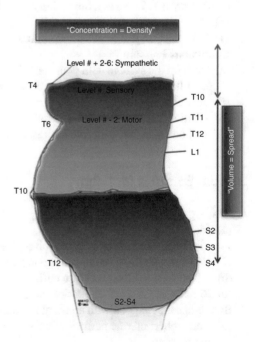

"Concentration = Density"

Level # + 2-6: Sympathetic
Level # : Sensory
Level # - 2: Motor

T4
T6
T10
T12

T10
T11
T12
L1

S2
S3
S4

S2-S4

"Volume = Spread"

Fig. 31.1 Diagram outlining the level of sensory blockade and drug dosing options when using an epidural for cesarean section

- Higher risk of airway edema from venous congestion, IV fluids, Pitocin → even if patient had a normal exam when epidural was first placed, still need to reexamine the airway. A Mallampati I may now be a Mallampati IV.
2. Always check dermatome level with ice before and after loading the epidural.
3. Always cycle the blood pressure cuff q5minutes when loading the epidural.
4. Epidural for non-emergent cesarean section
   - While briefing in the room, give 10 cc of 2% lidocaine with epinephrine 5 mcg/ml and bicarbonate.
   - When patient arrives in the OR and is lying flat, give another 5 cc of 2% lidocaine w/epi and bicarb until reaching goal T4 level.
5. Epidural for emergent cesarean section
   - 15–20 cc of 3% chloroprocaine.

Lower Extremity Motor Exam

- Hip flexion – L1, L2
- Knee extension – L3, L4
- Dorsiflexion of ankle, dorsiflexion of great toe – L5
- Plantarflexion of ankle – S1

A postpartum patient who underwent cesarean section using a lumbar spinal/epidural neuraxial technique now presents with foot drop. How do you rule out a neuraxial technique as the cause of the foot drop?

- Foot drop = inability to dorsiflex at the ankle
- If there were a spinal cord injury from the neuraxial anesthetic technique, there would also be inability to plantarflex the ankle.
- Isolated foot drop with no impairment of ankle plantarflexion is indicative of isolated peroneal nerve injury.
- Also consult neurology, electromyogram/nerve conduction studies (EMG/NCS) studies.

Continuous Spinal

32

Indications for Continuous Spinal rather than General Anesthesia

- Risk of general anesthesia outweighs risk of continuous spinal anesthetic
- Severe pulmonary disease
- Severe cardiac disease
  - Severe aortic stenosis
  - Severe mitral regurgitation
  - Severe pulmonary hypertension

Indications for Continuous Spinal rather than Single Shot Spinal

1. Severe cardiac disease
   (a) More severe hypotension and bradycardia based on how potently and how quickly you block the thoracic and lumbar spinal levels
      (i) Sympathetic fibers run from T1 to L2
   (b) Benefit of using isobaric rather than hyperbaric bupivacaine
      (i) Hyperbaric bupivacaine: more potent, spreads faster to reach more thoracic and lumbar levels, or settles in sacral region and does not provide intended dermatomal distribution.
      (ii) Isobaric bupivacaine: less of a sympathetic block, less hypotension, and keep the local anesthetic in the lumbar region.
   (c) Continuous spinals: enable the provider to titrate the local anesthetic, allowing the patient's body time to adjust
   (d) Single-shot spinals: all the local anesthetics are given at once, causing a large and fast sympathetic block
2. Severe pulmonary disease
   (a) "Pulmonary cripple" who is dependent on home oxygen

C. Sampankanpanich Soria et al., *Anesthesiology Resident Manual of Procedures*,
https://doi.org/10.1007/978-3-030-65732-1_32

(b) CO_2 retainer: indicated by elevated baseline HCO_3 on BMP
(c) Single-shot spinal: sudden blockade of nerve fibers innervating the intercostal muscles and other accessory muscles of respiration → significant loss in respiratory function → hypoventilation, CO_2 retention, and oxygen desaturation

Technique

- Same as regular spinal block but use an epidural kit
- 17 G epidural needle enters the dura and intrathecal space
  - Be prepared for a gush of CSF.
  - Have your epidural catheter ready to thread.
  - After removing the Touhy stylette with your right hand, quickly place your left thumb over the Touhy opening, being careful not to advance the Touhy needle.
- Thread 19 G epidural catheter. Warn patients that as the catheter is entering the intrathecal space, they may feel paresthesias in the lower extremities. This can be disconcerting to patients.
- Prior to threading the epidural catheter, 10 cc of preservative-free normal saline can be injected into the intrathecal space. Do NOT use sterile water, which is obviously hypotonic and contains benzyl alcohol preservative that is toxic to nerves.

How to Dose

- Name of the game is slow and gentle titration. You can always give more.
- Example loading doses: 0.5–1 cc increments of
  - 0.75% hyperbaric bupivacaine
  - 0.25% hypobaric bupivacaine
  - 0.5% isobaric bupivacaine
- Then titrate up to desired dermatome level with additional 0.5 cc of 0.75% hyperbaric bupivacaine.
- Re-dosing
  - If surgery duration is longer than 1–1.5 h, use 0.5 cc increments of 0.5% isobaric bupivacaine (about 1/3 to ½ the initial loading dose needed).

Why Aren't Continuous Spinal Catheters More Common?

- Concern for cauda equina syndrome
  - Historically associated with macrocatheters, which are no longer available in the United States.
  - Historically associated with 5% hyperbaric lidocaine, which is not used anymore intrathecally due to additional concern for toxic neurologic syndrome.

- Label these catheters carefully!
  - Other providers may mistake them for continuous epidural catheters
  - Epidural dosing in the intrathecal space → high spinal, cardiac and respiratory arrest

Intrathecal Narcotics

- Pros
  - Blocks pressure sensation in sacral region, sacral sparing S2–S4
  - Provides analgesic relief for 2–4 h
- Cons
  - Side effects include urinary retention, nausea/vomiting, pruritus, respiratory depression. If hydrophilic compound such as morphine is given, 12–24 h of monitoring is needed for signs of delayed respiratory depression.

Special Populations

- Elderly, male, with benign prostatic hypertrophy
- Prefer to avoid spinal anesthetic due to higher risk of urinary retention
- PACU protocol: bladder scan and straight catheterization if evidence of urinary retention
- Counsel patients to void when they go home, otherwise return within 12 h
- Balance risks of urinary retention with advantages of spinal anesthetic: severe cardiac disease, severe pulmonary disease, instrumentation of airway
- 1 in 4 patients with spinal block will have urinary retention when they go home – is this for sure and is it impacted by whether they went home before being allowed to void postop? This number seems high compared to when we do it right.

Combined Spinal-Epidurals

33

Indications for Combined Spinal-Epidural (CSEs)

1. Anticipated difficult, prolonged cesarean section
   (a) Multigravida
   (b) Multiparous
   (c) Obese
   (d) Prior abdominal/pelvic surgery with lots of scar tissue
2. For labor
   (a) To confirm epidural placement
   (b) To provide more immediate pain relief
      (i) Be selective: e.g., patients who are almost 10 cm dilated and will start to push. In the second stage of labor, the pain is somatic S2–S4. In the first stage of labor, the pain is visceral T10–L2, and a spinal is not needed.

Why Not to Do CSEs for Labor

1. You should not be doing CSEs to confirm a true LOR of your epidural. If you don't know where you are, don't put more things in.
2. To confirm true LOR, try threading the epidural catheter. The catheter will not thread in ligament.
3. By creating a dural puncture, you've increased the risk of postdural puncture headache.
4. You've theoretically increased the risk of infection because there is a hole in the dura and an epidural catheter is being placed just outside of it.

How to Place a CSE

1. Place epidural as you normally would.

© The Author(s), under exclusive license to Springer Nature Switzerland AG 2021
C. Sampankanpanich Soria et al., *Anesthesiology Resident Manual of Procedures*,
https://doi.org/10.1007/978-3-030-65732-1_33

2. Using a spinal needle that is longer than the length of the Touhy needle (check beforehand), advance until dural puncture is felt and obtain free flow of CSF.
3. Administer spinal dose of local anesthetic.
4. Remove spinal needle while carefully maintaining Touhy needle in same position.
5. Thread epidural catheter as quickly as possible.
6. Secure epidural catheter as normal.

How to Dose CSEs for Labor

- Up to 4 mg total of isobaric bupivacaine.
- E.g., 2–2.5 cc of 0.125% isobaric bupivacaine.
- Benefit of isobaric bupivacaine: stays where you've injected it. Gives you time to thread and secure your epidural.

Thoracic Epidurals

34

Benefits

- Cardiovascular: decreases postop MI, redistributes coronary blood flow, attenuates stress response and postoperative pain
- Pulmonary: superior analgesia, enables deep breathing exercises and early ambulation
- Gastrointestinal: facilitates return of bowel motility from improved pain control and decreased narcotic requirements; less constipation
- Improved postop analgesia and patient comfort
- Excellent for larger incisions across chest and abdomen
- Benefits less well established for minimally invasive procedures

Risks

- Close proximity of spinal cord
- Narrower epidural space
- Thinner ligamentum flavum
- Hypotension, nausea/vomiting, urinary retention
- Require personnel to manage on the floor

Insertion Technique

1. Identify landmarks
   (a) Spine of scapula is at level of T4
   (b) Inferior angle of scapula is at level of T7
   (c) Mid-thoracic spinous processes are more acutely angled
   (d) Laminae become more vertically oriented as move caudal
2. Insertion site target is T6–T8

© The Author(s), under exclusive license to Springer Nature Switzerland AG 2021   163
C. Sampankanpanich Soria et al., *Anesthesiology Resident Manual of Procedures*,
https://doi.org/10.1007/978-3-030-65732-1_34

3. Positioning the patient
   (a) Sitting or lateral decubitus position
   (b) Little benefit from exaggerated spinal flexion because thoracic facet joints mostly allow axillary rotation
   (c) Mayo stand/tray table at level of patient's shoulders to rest arms, can rest head down, and close eyes if more comfortable
4. IV sedation: small doses of midazolam 1–2 mg and fentanyl 25–50 mcg
5. Paramedian approach
   (a) Most common technique, easier than midline.
   (b) In thoracic spine, spinous processes are angulated and closely approximated; difficult to avoid bony obstruction when approaching from midline.
   (c) First identify bottom spinous process of intended interspace.
   (d) Insert local needle (use as finder needle) 1 cm lateral to the spinous process. Aim a little medial and caudal.
   (e) Goal is to hit lamina.
   (f) Once you hit lamina, advance the needle in and out, slowly walking the needle toward midline until you hit spinous process.
       (i) How do you know you've hit spinous process? Hit bone 2 cm shallower than lamina.
   (g) Numb the tract that the local needle takes.
   (h) Now repeat the same process using the Touhy needle.
   (i) Once you touch spinous process, walk the needle cephalad off of the spinous process until you enter interspinous ligament.
   (j) Remove stylette and screw on loss of resistance syringe.
   (k) Advance until loss of resistance (past interspinous ligament and ligamentum flavum) with air/saline.
   (l) Estimated distance to interspace = 1 cm + distance of Touhy where you hit lamina.
6. Midline approach
   (a) Needle must be advanced cephalad at a more acute angle to pass between the steep, down-sloping spinous processes.
   (b) Longer path for needle to travel than paramedian approach due to the steep angle.
   (c) Easy to do in thin patients with prominent spinous processes.
7. Tips
   (a) Do not inject too much saline. The epidural space is small. It quickly becomes difficult to palpate landmarks.
   (b) If you don't hit lamina, try a new insertion site 1 cm cephalad or caudad.

Wet Taps and Epidural Blood Patches

35

Common Scenarios

1. Traumatic lumbar puncture (Table 35.1)
2. Wet tap = intrathecal placement of Touhy needle during intended epidural placement (Table 40.2)
   (a) Thoracic epidural for pain management
   (b) Labor epidural for obstetric anesthesia
3. Intrathecal contrast injection for CT scans

Risk Factors

Indications for Blood Patch

1. Failed conservative treatment (IV fluids, caffeine, fioricet, NSAIDs)
2. Headache preventing patient from performing activities of daily living
   (a) Unable to work or go to school
   (b) Unable to care for newborn baby

Table 35.1 Risk factors for wet taps

High risk	Low risk
Young: big intervertebral spaces, larger CSF leaks	Old: fibrosis and ossification of spine; tighter, smaller intervertebral spaces; smaller CSF leak
Thin	Overweight/obese
Large bore needle	Small bore needle
Cutting needle (17 G Tuohy needle)	Pencil needle (25 G spinal needle)

Contraindications to Blood Patch

1. Febrile
2. History of bacteremia without negative blood culture
3. PDPH vs. meningitis, nuchal rigidity

Diagnosing Post-dural Puncture Headache

1. History of known or suspected wet tap
2. Typically frontal headache and can be all over the head
3. Position: worse with sitting or standing; only relief from lying down

What to Do if You Wet Tap a Patient

1. Remove the Touhy needle and go to a different location for the procedure.
2. After the procedure, tell the patient what happened.
    (a) Counsel the patient about 50% (no longer 1 in 100) risk of post-dural puncture headache.
3. Remove labor epidural 2–3 h after delivery.
4. Conservative measures: oral and IV hydration, caffeine, Fioricet (caffeine-acetaminophen tablets), and oral analgesics.
5. If conservative measures fail, consider epidural blood patch.

Does Wet Tap = Post-dural Puncture Headache?

- CSF production = 500 cc/day
    - Absorbed by arachnoid villi
    - Produced by fourth ventricle ependymal cells
- Cause of headache
    - Dural leak → pull on meninges
    - Cerebral vasodilation to refill space create by CSF loss
    - Caffeine treatment:
      Vasoconstricts cerebral blood vessels
      Stimulates ependymal cells to make CSF
- Larger the dural puncture, greater the CSF leak, greater the likelihood of post-dural puncture headache
    - 1 in 100 with 25 G spinal needle vs. 1 in 2 with 17 G Touhy needle; risk increases with multiple attempts

When to Do a Blood Patch

- Not done immediately after a wet tap on laboring patient
- Laboring patient will strain, bear down → dislodge blood patch
- Try conservative treatment for a few days first

How to Counsel Patient About Epidural Blood Patch

1. If patient had wet tap previously, may have a wet tap again while trying to do the blood patch.
2. Should have pain relief within 30–60 min of the procedure.
3. Requires placement of a new sterile IV.
4. Risks
   (a) Bleeding
   (b) Infection
   (c) Nerve injury
   (d) 1 in 100 headache
   (e) Lower back pain radiating down back and buttocks
   (f) Cauda equine syndrome = purposefully creating an epidural hematoma

Blood Patch Technique

1. Equipment Needed
   (a) Peripheral IV
       (i) Tourniquet
       (ii) Mayo stand or tray table for patient to rest arm
       (iii) Sterile blue towels
       (iv) Sterile gloves
       (v) Chloraprep
       (vi) 10 cc syringes
       (vii) Stopcock
       (viii) 18 G catheters
   (b) Standard epidural kit
   (c) Second provider ideal, one provider only is possible
2. Positioning
   (a) Ideally sitting
   (b) Supine, lateral decubitus possible

3. Two-provider technique
   (a) First provider places a new, sterile PIV.
       (i) To prevent leakage of blood from PIV, attach stopcock to IV catheter
           and close stopcock to patient while awaiting epidural securement.
       (ii) When requested, draws blood off of PIV using stopcock and 10 cc
           syringe and carefully passes syringe of blood to second provider.
   (b) Second provider enters epidural space with Touhy needle and injects blood.
       (i) Maximum, total amount of blood: 30 cc.
       (ii) Give 5 cc at a time until patient reports a backache.
       (iii) Pause until backache resolves.
       (iv) Then give 1 cc at a time.
       (v) Stop completely when backache recurs.
4. One-provider technique
   (a) Provider places tourniquet on patient's arm and preps and drapes the arm
       sterilely for eventual PIV placement.
   (b) Provider walks over to patient's back and places epidural.
   (c) Provider walks around to patient's front and places PIV with stopcock.
   (d) Provider draws off 10 cc of blood and walks to back of patient, injects blood
       into epidural space.

Total Intravenous Anesthetics

36

Indications for TIVA

1. Malignant hyperthermia
   (a) Requires complete avoidance of all volatile anesthetics
2. Surgery on the vocal cords or the tracheobronchial tree
   (a) Inhaled anesthetic would be released into the environment, and all staff members would be exposed
   (b) Examples: flexible bronchoscopy, rigid bronchoscopy, "shared airway"
3. Severe postoperative nausea and vomiting
   (a) Avoid all inhaled anesthetics completely, nitrous oxide, and volatiles
   (b) Propofol has antiemetic properties
4. Elevated intracranial pressure (ICP)
   (a) Neurosurgery cases where even with "0.5 MAC" or less of volatile anesthetic, still encountering elevated ICP, high risk herniation, "tight brain," poor operating conditions for surgeons
5. Neuromonitoring
   (a) Neuromonitoring indicates motor-evoked potentials (MEP), somatosensory-evoked potentials (SSEP) signal interference despite balanced anesthetic
6. Decrease environmental exposure
7. Power outage, equipment availability
   (a) No ventilator
   (b) No volatile agents

Goals of Anesthesia

1. Amnesia
2. Analgesia
3. Muscle relaxation

© The Author(s), under exclusive license to Springer Nature Switzerland AG 2021   169
C. Sampankanpanich Soria et al., *Anesthesiology Resident Manual of Procedures*,
https://doi.org/10.1007/978-3-030-65732-1_36

What Drugs Can Be Used for TIVA?

- TIVA is best for cases <2.5–3 h.
- Every medication has a half-life. The longer the medication is running, the greater the context-sensitive half-life, the trickier it becomes to have timely wake-ups. Medications must be gradually titrated down based on estimated steady-state to allow for a smooth emergence.

I. Propofol
   (a) Pros:
       (i) Amnestic properties, some muscle relaxation, antiemetic properties
   (b) Cons:
       (i) No analgesic properties
       (ii) Context-sensitive half-life increases over time
       (iii) Need to titrate down during the case
       (iv) General guidelines: If run for >3 h, will need to discontinue at least 45 min prior to intended wake-up.
   (c) Fun fact: Infusion pumps are available in Europe that automatically titrate infusion rate based on targeted concentration and patient height/body weight, pre-programmed into pump settings. Pump automatically estimates plasma concentration of propofol over time. Unfortunately, these are not available in the United States.

II. Ketamine
   (a) Five mechanisms of action
       (i) Anti-NMDA → analgesia
       (ii) Muscarinic → increased airway secretions
       (iii) Mu receptors → pain control
       (iv) Calcium channel receptors → direct myocardial depression
       (v) Adrenals → increased catecholamine release
   (b) Goal is to stay below a total dose of 1–2 mg/kg for the entire case
       (i) Caution with units on pump settings: ketamine 5 mcg/kg/min = 0.005 mg/kg/min (on the pump settings) = 0.3 mg/kg/h (in EPIC)
   (c) Pros:
       (i) Analgesic and amnestic properties
       (ii) Typically maintains spontaneous ventilation, but at higher doses can make patient apneic especially with concomitant opioid administration
       (iii) Decreases opiate requirements postoperatively
   (d) Cons:
       (i) Hallucinations, disassociation, recommended to give midazolam before starting ketamine or to smooth emergence after ketamine
       (ii) Indirectly increases sympathetic activity → hypertension, tachycardia
       (iii) Direct myocardial depressant
       (iv) Increases bronchosecretions → increased risk of laryngospasm. Need to give glycopyrrolate in advance to dry the airway

III. Fentanyl
  (a) Context-sensitive half-life increases over time
  (b) Need to titrate down or will prolong wake-up
  (c) Not a good narcotic to run as an infusion (provider preference)
IV. Remifentanil
  (a) Degraded by plasma esterases.
  (b) Context-sensitive half-life does not change over time.
  (c) Short half-life, stops working 3–5 min after discontinued as long as you're using recommended doses – at higher doses remifentanil effects may persist for longer than usual.
  (d) Need to titrate long-acting narcotic like fentanyl once getting patient breathing.
  (e) Debate over causing hyperalgesia vs. provider forgetting to titrate in long-acting narcotic before waking patient up.

Awareness Under Anesthesia

- Downside to TIVA is that there is no display equivalent to MAC for IV medications → don't know how deep a patient is.
- Particularly dangerous if patient is paralyzed.
- How to assess awareness:
  - BIS monitor: goal BIS number is <40 and low signal activity tracing
  - Neuromonitoring during neurosurgery: assess cerebral activity and level of burst suppression on EEG.
- Ideally have access to the PIV that is running the TIVA. Check this PIV at least q15–20 min during the case to ensure it is not infiltrated or leaking. Ideally have the IV site and IV tubing visible to you at all times.
  - Nightmare scenario: patient is paralyzed, PIV infiltrated, and TIVA is leaking subcutaneous into patient's limb or all over the floor.
- If patient has sudden increase in heart rate or blood pressure, it is difficult to know if this is due to patient awareness or pain, especially if patient is paralyzed. Careful evaluation is warranted.

Example TIVA Technique

1. Medications
  (a) Alaris pump with 4 channels
  (b) Normal saline carrier (50–100 ml/h): ensures constant forward flow
  (c) Remifentanil 0.1–0.2 mcg/kg/min (2–4 mg diluted in a 100 cc bag of NS)
  (d) Propofol 100 mcg/kg/min (use 100 ml bottles)
  (e) Phenylephrine 10–20 mcg/min (10 mg diluted in 100 cc bag of NS)
  (f) Put the TIVA infusion on a solo IV, so TIVA meds are not being bolused each time other medications or fluids are administered.

2. TIVA-style induction
    (a) Pre-oxygenate patient and position for intubation.
    (b) Connect TIVA tubing to patient's PIV and start the carrier, remifentanil 0.1 mcg/kg/min, and propofol 100 mcg/kg/min.
    (c) Do not give any additional propofol, just paralytic for intubation, and fentanyl 50–100 mcg.
3. Maintenance
    (a) Keep an eye on the clock and the pace of the surgeons.
    (b) Propofol infusion
        (i) Goal with propofol infusion is to achieve a constant steady-state, so decrease propofol infusion by 5 mcg/kg/min q30min.
        (ii) After the first 30 min, decrease the propofol infusion to 95 mcg/kg/min.
        (iii) 30 min later (1 h into the case), decrease the propofol infusion to 90 mcg/kg/min.
        (iv) 30 min later (1.5 h into the case), decrease the propofol infusion to 85 mcg/kg/min.
        (v) 30 min later (2 h into the case), decrease the propofol infusion to 80 mcg/kg/min.
        (vi) For the remainder of the case, continue the propofol at 80 mcg/kg/min until start to reach closure.
        (vii) Do NOT bolus with propofol. Will delay wakeup.
        (viii) Do NOT increase the propofol gtt. Will increase context-sensitive half-life with dose and duration. Won't know half-life.
    (c) Remifentanil infusion
        (i) As needed for periods of increased surgical stimulation or if the patient does not have adequate pain control.
        (ii) Use the remifentanil as a bridge until longer-acting narcotic like fentanyl can be given.
        (iii) Use remifentanil because context-sensitive half-life is short and doesn't change. Short duration of action.
        (iv) Bolus remifentanil 0.25–0.5 mcg/kg and titrate fentanyl 25–50 mcg.
4. Emergence
    (a) When surgeons start closing, decrease propofol gtt to 50 mcg/kg/min and continue to monitor for signs of light anesthesia.
    (b) Continue the remifentanil gtt.
    (c) Turn off the propofol completely at least 10–15 min prior to extubation.
    (d) Must watch the surgeons very carefully for timing.
    (e) When patient is spontaneously breathing, titrate in fentanyl boluses 25 mcg at a time to goal $ETCO_2$ 50, RR 8–10.
    (f) If patient lightens too early, bolus with remifentanil 0.25–0.5 mcg/kg, not propofol, and give a little more fentanyl 25 mcg.
    (g) Patients move before they remember.

Monitored Anesthesia Care

37

Rules of Thumb

1. Every anesthetic is an MAC. We provide a service: preoperative, intraoperative, and postoperative.
2. Always anticipate the anesthetic going one level deeper than planned (Table 40.3).
3. Always be prepared to convert to general anesthesia.
4. You "shall" monitor $ETCO_2$. Exceptions:
    (a) Cardiopulmonary bypass
    (b) Magnetic field and cannot have monitor
    (c) Equipment malfunctions intraoperatively

Indications for MAC/Sedation

- Patient preference for regional/neuraxial/local anesthetic infiltration rather than general anesthesia
- Avoid hemodynamic changes of general anesthesia
    - Severe cardiac disease
- Avoid instrumenting the airway, paralyzing patient, and losing pharyngeal tone
    - Difficult intubation
    - Severe pulmonary disease

Ideal Patient

- Comfortable: adequate analgesia from regional nerve block, neuraxial block, or local anesthetic infiltration of surgical field
- Cooperative, calm, psychological buy-in

© The Author(s), under exclusive license to Springer Nature Switzerland AG 2021   173
C. Sampankanpanich Soria et al., *Anesthesiology Resident Manual of Procedures*,
https://doi.org/10.1007/978-3-030-65732-1_37

- Communication: challenging with language barrier, intellectual disability, psychiatric disease, intoxicated/substance abuse
- Airway not far away from anesthesiologist in case of airway obstruction

Anesthetic Techniques

I. Propofol
   (a) Use: FDA Guidelines
      (i) 100–150 mcg/kg/min for 3–5 min, then...
      (ii) 25–75 mcg/kg/min for 5–10 min, then...
      (iii) 25–50 mcg/kg/min for remainder of case
      (iv) OR 0.5 mg/kg initial bolus, then switch to infusion
      (v) Recommended to be done by infusion, not by bolus, to decrease risk of respiratory and cardiac arrest with boluses
   (b) Pros
      (i) Most commonly used drug for MAC/sedation.
      (ii) Widely available.
      (iii) Fast-acting, effective.
      (iv) Can go from 0% to 100%: mild sedation/awake to total general anesthesia with propofol alone.
      (v) Antiemetic properties
   (c) Cons
      (i) Eventually with enough propofol, will become apneic.
      (ii) Everyone obstructs their airway eventually.
      (iii) At higher levels of infusion rate and longer duration of infusion (>2–2.5 h), the context-sensitive half-life increases.
      (iv) Burns on administration.
         1. Give fentanyl or lidocaine (let sit in PIV)
II. Dexmedetomidine (Precedex)
   (a) Use
      (i) Infusion 0.3–0.7 mcg/kg/h
      (ii) Bolus 0.5 mcg/kg – administer over 10 min
      (iii) Watch for bradycardia, hypotension with bolus due to alpha-2 agonist effects
      (iv) Turn off ~30 min prior to surgical closure
   (b) Pros
      (i) Maintain spontaneous ventilation regardless of the dose
      (ii) Patient awake
      (iii) Basically the infusion is equivalent of clonidine because both have alpha-2 agonist effects
      (iv) Some analgesia
      (v) Great for awake fiberoptic intubation because of maintenance of spontaneous ventilation but patient is sedated and comfortable

    (c) Cons
        (i) Onset of action 10–15 min
            1. Bolus in pre-operative room or tell surgeon you need 15 min to reach a good level of sedation (can prep and drape during that time).
        (ii) Hypotension, bradycardia if given too quickly
            1. Also reports of hypertension
        (iii) Duration of action is >2–3 h, even though patient is awake and breathing, so not ideal for outpatient surgery when patient will go home.
        (iv) Cannot deepen to general anesthesia, no matter how much uptitration.
        (v) Patient awake, not asleep. Not good if having anxious patient who is moving around. Would need to supplement with additional medication like propofol.

III. Ketamine
    (a) Use
        (i) Maintenance dose: 1–5 mcg/kg/min
        (ii) Not routinely used as the sole anesthetic agent
    (b) Pros
        (i) Really good analgesia
            1. Example 1: nerve block not working well, want to avoid converting to general anesthetic
            2. Example 2: pregnant patient's spinal block wearing off, about to finish closing during a cesarean section
        (ii) Maintain spontaneous ventilation, but also at higher doses if needed, can become general anesthesia on ketamine alone
    (c) Cons
        (i) Emergence delirium, disassociation: patient doesn't understand the difference between reality and their vivid hallucinations. Recommended to give midazolam for amnesia and anxiolysis *before* giving ketamine.
        (ii) Increases HR and BP (may be a PRO)
        (iii) At high enough dose, patient will become apneic
        (iv) Direct myocardial depressant

Airway Management

- Goal is to maintain spontaneous ventilation
- Risk factors for airway obstruction
  - Oversedation: combination of hypnotics, benzodiazepines, and narcotics
  - H/o obstructive sleep apnea
  - Obese
- Tips and tricks
  - Use simple face mask or nasal cannula with $ETCO_2$ monitoring.
  - $ETCO_2$ is your friend!
  - Establish level of sedation early on while surgeons are prepping patient.

- Once patient is deep enough, empirically insert a nasal trumpet lubricated with lidocaine ointment.
- Position patient well using foam donut and towels for head extension.
- When patient obstructs, try verbal stimulation: gently ask patient to take deep breaths. Do not startle patient; if patient moves, surgeon will not be happy.
- If patient does not respond to verbal stimulation, provide gentle chin lift, and jaw thrust if needed.

Conversion to General Anesthesia

- Always have rescue airways available
  - Blade and ETT
  - LMA
- Fastest is to pre-oxygenate, induce with propofol 2 mg/kg, and insert LMA.

Emergence Without Nitrous Oxide

38

Instructions

1. As soon as possible, given the surgical conditions, reverse neuromuscular blockade.
2. Get the patient breathing on their own by using synchronized intermittent mandatory ventilation (SIMV) or pressure support ventilation (PSVPro). Ventilation goals:
   (a) Patient initiates all of their own breaths.
   (b) Minimal pressure support of 5 cmH$_2$O.
   (c) Trigger flow of 2 L/min.
   (d) ETCO$_2$ of 50.
   (e) RR 8–10.
3. Turn down the sevoflurane. Goal is for the end-tidal sevoflurane to be 0 as soon as possible.
4. To ensure lack of awareness while patient is breathing off sevoflurane:
   (a) Give propofol 20–30 mg q10 min (dose titrated to patient tolerance) OR
   (b) Use propofol gtt 25–50 mcg/kg/min but discontinue 10 min prior to extubation
5. To ensure analgesia:
   (a) Give fentanyl 25 mcg at a time, titrated to ETCO$_2$ 50 and RR 8–10.
   (b) If a patient breathes at a faster rate to a lower ETCO$_2$ than this while still under anesthesia, they will breathe even faster when awake. This indicates that the patient's pain is poorly controlled.
6. Signs that patient is in pain, the anesthetic is too light, and/or the patient will move/awaken too early
   (a) Tachypnea
   (b) Low ETCO$_2$
   (c) Sigh breaths
   (d) Irregular respiratory pattern
   (e) Tachycardia
   (f) Hypertension
   (g) Sweating

C. Sampankanpanich Soria et al., *Anesthesiology Resident Manual of Procedures*, https://doi.org/10.1007/978-3-030-65732-1_38

Craniotomies

39

What Is Wrong with Nitrous Oxide?

- Controversial topic
- Personal preference
- Use varies by institution
- Pros
  - Less hypotension compared to volatile anesthetics → intravascularly depleted, hypotensive/bradycardic patient
  - Quick onset of action
  - Short duration of action (5 min) does not saturate fat/muscle as much as volatile anesthetics → faster emergence
  - Odorless → gentler inhalation induction for children
- Cons
  - Fills up air-filled cavities quickly → common contraindications: bowel obstruction, pneumothorax, increased intra-ocular pressure
  - Distends bowel → suboptimal operating conditions for surgeons working in abdomen
  - Decreases FiO_2
  - Inactivates vitamin B12

General Set-Up for Craniotomy

1. Induction/intubation with table already turned 180°.
   (a) Decreases time to turn bed and untangle lines.
   (b) Practicing for emergency craniotomies.
2. Second PIV in the foot

C. Sampankanpanich Soria et al., *Anesthesiology Resident Manual of Procedures*,
https://doi.org/10.1007/978-3-030-65732-1_39

3. ± Central line, depending on the case
   (a) Discuss site placement with surgeon
   (b) Generally internal jugular CVCs are contraindicated → obstruct cerebral venous drainage → increases ICP
   (c) Traditionally prefer subclavian CVC or peripherally inserted line (e.g., from antecubital or basilica vein), but femoral CVC also acceptable
4. ± Multiorifice catheter, depending on the case
5. Radial or pedial arterial line
   (a) Pre-induction if high risk of hemorrhaging during induction (e.g., ruptured aneurysm).
   (b) Post-induction otherwise (most patients, more comfortable).
6. Bair Hugger
   (a) Consider permissive hypothermia to help decrease $CMRO_2$ and therefore ICP.
   (b) Minimum temperature is 35 C.
   (c) Goal T 35–37 C during case.
   (d) Rewarm to 36–67 C by emergence, otherwise will delay wake-up.
   (e) If coagulopathic, do not do permissive hypothermia.
7. Esophageal temperature probe
8. Two soft bite blocks between the molars
   (a) Confirm placement with a second provider and document this.
   (b) Do not want patient to bite tongue while running motors on facial nerves.
9. Taping the eyes
   (a) Silk tape the eyes closed after induction, before intubation, so do not scratch corneas.
   (b) Surgeons remove silk tape to do brain mapping.
   (c) Prior to surgeons' prepping the skin, place half-small tegaderms over the eyes so skin prep does not leak under eyelids and burn corneas.
10. Circuit extension
    (a) Do not forget to use extra-long circuits or put extensions on the Y piece.
    (b) Put extension tubing on the green bag.
    (c) Use straight connector to connect ETT to circuit. Right-angle connector tents the drape up, bothers the surgeon.
11. Airway/A-line tray
    (a) Leave at new head of bed 180.
12. Bed remote
    (a) Test the remote before the surgeons start!
    (b) Bed may be reversed. Put labeled stickers so you know the maneuvers of each button.
13. Arterial blood gases
    (a) General good rule of thumb: check q1h
    (b) General goals: Na WNL, glucose 100–200
        (i) For the injured brain, hyperglycemia is just as bad as hypoglycemia.

Drugs to Prepare

- Standard drugs
  - Propofol 20 cc × 2
  - Rocuronium 10 cc × 1
  - Succinylcholine 10 cc × 1
  - Ephedrine 10 cc
  - Phenylephrine 10 cc
  - Lidocaine 5 cc × 3
      Induction
      Head pinning
      Head un-pinning
  - Labetalol
  - Fentanyl 20 cc
  - NO MIDAZOLAM!!!
  - Abx: usually cefazolin 1–2 g
- Drug on standby
  - Nicardipine gtt and bolus
- Alaris pump × 2 with at least 6 channels
  - Normal saline carrier at 50–100 cc/h
  - Propofol gtt (100 cc bottle)
  - Remifentanil gtt (2–4 mg diluted in 100 cc NS)
  - Phenylephrine gtt (10 mg diluted in 100 cc NS)
- Extra drugs to have available on surgeon request
  - Dexamethasone 4–8 mg
      Do not give for traumatic brain injury
  - Keppra (Levetiracetam) 1000 mg in 100 cc bag
  - Mannitol 20% (200 mg/ml)
      Infuse on pump over 30 min
      Separate line/port so it does not clot your infusions
  - Lasix 10 mg/ml
  - Hypertonic saline (3% NaCl)
- Crystalloid
  - 2 × 1 L bags of NS or Plasmalyte on fluid warmers
  - Varies by provider preference and institutional availability
  - Normal saline (0.9% NaCl)
      pH 5
      154 mEq/L Na
      154 mEq/L Cl
      308 mEq/L osmolarity
  - Plasmalyte
      pH 7.4
      140 mEq/L Na

  98 mEq/L Cl
  5 mEq/L K
  3 mEq/L Mg
  27 mEq/L acetate
  23 mEq/L gluconate
  296 mEq/L osmolarity
- Goal: maintain normal serum sodium. Hyponatremia → cerebral edema, increased ICP, poor surgical operating conditions.

Anesthetic Plan Without Nitrous Oxide

1. Induction
   (a) *Maximum* amount of fentanyl for the *entire* case is 50–100 mcg.
       (i) The sleepier / less responsive a patient is prior to induction, the less fentanyl given.
       (ii) *No* long-acting narcotic such as dilaudid.
   (b) Lidocaine 1 mg/kg
       (i) Blunts sympathetic response to intubation
       (ii) Decreases ICP
   (c) Propofol 2 mg/kg
   (d) Rocuronium or succinylcholine – dose depends on routine versus RSI
2. Intubation
   (a) Gentle direct laryngoscopy → avoid overstimulation → sympathetic response.
   (b) Quick control of airway, avoid hypercapnia → increased ICP.
3. Maintenance
   (a) There is no narcotic load on board.
   (b) Will not be starting nitrous oxide to speed uptake of volatile anesthetic.
   (c) As soon as ETT is secured, connect infusions to patient and press start.
       (i) 0.5 MAC sevoflurane – for awareness
       (ii) Propofol 100 mcg/kg/min → rapidly titrate down to 25 mcg/kg/min for PONV prophylaxis
       (iii) Remifentanil 0.1–0.2 mcg/kg/min
   (d) Less stimulation after dura is opened
       (i) The parts of the brain that feel pain are the blood vessels.
   (e) Do not paralyze patient. No need. Surgeons do not need muscle relaxations. Neuromonitoring may be checking MEPs.
4. Emergence
   (a) Discontinue propofol gtt as soon as possible.
   (b) Carefully but quickly wean off sevoflurane.
       (i) Keep careful eye on speed of surgical closure.
   (c) Continue remifentanil gtt until the end.
       (i) May need to go as high as 0.3 mcg/kg/min.

(d) When pins are removed, d/c remifentanil gtt or titrate down. Estimate time for head wrapping → jostle head and ETT → stimulates the patient to cough.

(e) No pain, no gain.

Anesthetic Plan with Nitrous Oxide

1. Induction
    (a) Narcotic load: fentanyl titrated to apnea (for cases at least 4 h long; if shorter, still do narcotic load but do not need to go apneic).
        (i) Method #1: empirically give 500 mcg up front, then titrate more.
        (ii) Method #2: truly titrate fentanyl. Onset of action 6 min.
        (iii) Calmly call patient's name verbally, ask them to open eyes, give thumbs up.
        (iv) Goal: patient apneic, nonresponsive to verbal stimuli.
        (v) How you induce is how you awaken.
    (b) Lidocaine 1 mg/kg
    (c) Propofol 0.5–1 mg/kg
        (i) Don't need much once have narcotic load
    (d) Rocuronium or succinylcholine – dose depends on routine versus RSI
2. Intubation
    (a) Gentle direct laryngoscopy → avoid overstimulation → sympathetic response.
    (b) Quick control of airway, avoid hypercapnia → increased ICP.
3. Maintenance
    (a) Inhaled anesthetics: 2/1 N_2O/O_2 and 0.5 MAC sevoflurane.
    (b) Augment blood pressure with phenylephrine gtt as needed.
    (c) Remifentanil gtt as needed, but already have big narcotic load, will last for >4 h case.
    (d) Fentanyl gtt
        (i) Provider preference
        (ii) 2 mcg/kg/h until dura is open
        (iii) Once dura is opened, 1 mcg/kg/h
        (iv) When surgeons done with brain, turn off
    (e) Paralysis
        (i) Contraindicated if neuromonitoring is checking MEPs
        (ii) Maintain in reversible state: 1–2 twitches maximum until head dressing is done
    (f) Avoid propofol as much as possible as a maintenance drug, unless TIVA required (neuromonitoring poor signals; tight brain, high ICP).
    (g) Head pinning
        (i) Watch surgeons carefully at start of case!!!
        (ii) Watch your ETT when surgeons lift/rotate head

      (iii) Propofol, fentanyl, and lidocaine in line in preparation for head pinning
      (iv) Variable methods
        1. Empirically give propofol 50 mg prior to head pinning
        2. Give 100 mg lidocaine 2 min prior to head pinning
        3. Empirically give ½ induction dose of fentanyl prior to head pinning
      (v) Do not overshoot → fighting hypotension

4. Emergence
   (a) When surgeons are done with the brain, turn off sevoflurane and run on as much N_2O as possible.
   (b) Titrate long-acting antihypertensive such as labetalol to avoid hypertension on emergence.
   (c) If during emergence, you think the patient needs more narcotic, use remifentanil gtt and discontinue 3–5 min before emergence.
   (d) Crucial that when running such a light anesthetic, patient stays paralyzed. Movement while in head pins → disaster.
   (e) Head un-pinning
       (i) Lidocaine 100 mg again
   (f) When head dressing is on, turn off nitrous oxide completely and run 100% oxygen at high flows.
   (g) Do not reverse patient until head pins are removed. Continue over-breathing patient on SIMV mode.
   (h) Gently remove OG tube and temperature probe. Suction oropharynx with the OG tube (softer than Yankauer).
   (i) Deflate ETT cuff and reinflate because nitrous oxide accumulates in the cuff. High pressure in cuff stimulates patient.
   (j) Do not let anyone touch the patient! Surgeons get restless and start opening eyelids and sternal rubbing. No one touches the patient. Startled patient = high ICP.
   (k) Start verbally stimulating patient once nitrous oxide is less than 10–14%.
   (l) As soon as patient opens eyes and takes a breath, pull the ETT. It is early, risk laryngospasm, but prevents coughing and elevated ICP.

Neuro Exam While Intubated, Immediately Postop

- On a remifentanil infusion of 0.1 mcg/kg/min, an intubated patient can usually perform a cognitive exam and tolerate an ETT.

Multiorifice Catheter

- Indications for placement?
  - High risk of venous air embolism
    Posterior fossa near confluence of sinuses

 - Empirical placement prior to start of surgery
     Ready to use
     High-risk situation
 - Placement after VAE occurs
     Less time, unprepared, during a resuscitation
     Suboptimal patient positioning
- Purpose of multiorifice catheter?
  - Rapidly extract large volumes of air from the RA, breaking the "air lock" that causes loss of cardiac output.
  - Even under controlled ideal situations, success rate is 30–60%.
  - Catheter can migrate with position change.
- Which catheter to use?
  - Large bore 14 G, single lumen, multiorifice catheters have done best in human and animal studies.
  - Ideally placed via R subclavian access.
  - Shorter, direct access to the R atrium than other points of entry.
  - Avoid IJ placement of lines in general for cranis to prevent blockage of venous drainage, increased ICP.
- Where to place the catheter?
  - Ideal location is tip of catheter 2 cm past the junction of the SVC and the RA.
- How to confirm location?
  - TEE
  - Radiograph – CXR intraop after placement
  - Intravascular EKG
      Normally it has an electrode built into it that you hook up to your white lead, the RA lead of your 3 or 5-lead EKG.
      Flush the lumen w/ $NaHCO_3$ to reduce electrical impedance.
      Catheter advanced into the RV, detected by transducing the pressure waveform.
      Withdraw the catheter until have biphasic p wave (mid-atrium) and then further back until p wave and QRS complex are of the same amplitude.
      Then pull back 1 cm and secure.

Hyperventilation and ICP

- $CO_2 + H_2O \Leftrightarrow H^+ + HCO_3^-$
- Hyperventilation → low $PaCO_2$ → high pH → cerebral vasoconstriction
- Why does hyperventilation to decrease ICP only work in the short term?
  - Only works for a few hours. Over time, the brain/CSF alters itself to move protons into the CSF and lower the pH. So, relatively speaking, the pH normalizes on its own.
- What do you do if you pick up a patient from the ICU to go to the OR for craniotomy and the patient's current ventilator settings are to hyperventilate?

- If you suddenly "normo-ventilate" the patient, there will be an acute rise in CO_2, but the brain is still pumping H+ into the CSF. Now there will be an acute drop in the pH and a resultant cerebral vasodilation.
- Why is it important to secure the airway as fast as possible when worried about ICP?
  - In the apneic patient, $ETCO_2$ rises by 6 in the first minute, and then 3 mmHg/min for every minute thereafter.

Mannitol

- Always double-check with the surgeons before administering. May request mannitol before or after dural opening.
- Typical dosing is 0.5–2 g/kg. Administer over at least 30 min.
- Give in separate infusion port or IV. May clot off IV line.
- At cold temperatures, the medication will crystallize.
- Creates an osmotic gradient → fluid shift from intracellular to extracellular space → temporarily increases effective circulating volume → osmotic diuresis. Caution in heart failure patients.

Hypertonic Saline (3% NaCl)

- Typical dosing for cerebral edema is 3–5 cc/kg over 10–20 min.
- 3 cc/kg of hypertonic saline will increase plasma Na by 2–3 mmol/L.
- Check serum Na regularly. Caution with dramatic rises in Na.

Liver Transplants

40

Drugs

Extra Equipment (*institutional variation, often run by perfusionist) (Table 40.1)

1. Belmont Machine
2. Arterial Blood Gas analyzer/iSTAT

Blood Products

1. Designated fridge in the OR for blood (Tables 40.3 and 40.4)
2. Verify with OR RN that hospital blood bank has been notified of liver transplant.
3. Double check that PRBCs, FFP, and platelets (10 + 10 + 2) will be in the room by the time dissection begins.
4. Order cryoprecipitate if needed (not automatically part of the massive transfusion protocol).

Monitors and Lines

1. Routine ASA monitors
2. Radial arterial line ± awake, depends on underlying cardiac and pulmonary function
   (a) Example: severe aortic stenosis, severe pulmonary hypertension
3. Femoral arterial line
4. Right Internal Jugular Vein (IJ) (RIJ) large bore central line, ± left Internal Jugular Vein (IJ) (LIJ) large bore central line
   (a) Option 1: Double stick: 2 × Cordises in R IJ
   (b) Option 2: 1 R IJ Cordis +1 L J Cordis

© The Author(s), under exclusive license to Springer Nature Switzerland AG 2021
C. Sampankanpanich Soria et al., *Anesthesiology Resident Manual of Procedures*,
https://doi.org/10.1007/978-3-030-65732-1_40

Table 40.1 Common medications organized by action to have prepared when performing a liver transplant

Narcotics	Midazolam 10 cc
	Fentanyl 20 cc
Induction agents	Etomidate 10 cc
	Propofol 20 cc
Paralytic	Succinylcholine 10 cc
	Rocuronium 10 cc
Steroids	Methylprednisolone 500 mg × 1 (at beginning and end of case)
Antibiotics	Ampicillin-sulbactam 3 g
Uppers (inotropes, pressors)	Ephedrine 10 cc syringe
	Phenylephrine 10 cc syringe
	Epinephrine gtt (pre-program to 0.02 mcg/kg/min)
	Phenylephrine gtt (pre-program to 20 mcg/min)
	Norepinephrine gtt (pre-program to 1 mg/min)
Downers (antihypertensives)	Nicardipine gtt (pre-program to 1 mg/h)
	Nitroglycerin gtt (pre-program to 20 mcg/min)
Emergency drugs	Vasopressin 1 unit/ml
*Most institutions have a	Epinephrine 10 mcg/ml in 10 cc syringe
designated "Anesthesia Liver	Epinephrine 1 mg/10 ml in 10 cc syringe
Cart" containing these drugs	Atropine 1 mg/10 ml in 10 cc syringe
	Lidocaine 100 mg/10 ml in 10 cc syringe
	*Calcium chloride 1000 mg/10 ml in 10 cc syringe
	*Sodium bicarbonate 50 meq/50 ml in 50 ml syringe
	*MULTIPLE boxes stacked on top of the anesthesia cart/machine very close by
Fluids	500 cc bottles of albumin
	100 cc and 250 cc bags of normal saline to dilute medications
	1 L bags of normal saline spiked and on fluid warmers

    (c) Option 3: 14/16 G PIV + R IJ Cordis

    (d) 1 central line is for Belmont machine

5. ± Swan Ganz catheter

    (a) Risks of PA catheter: atrial or ventricular arrhythmias, clot formation, traumatic placement

    (b) Benefits of catheter: assess hemodynamic changes, volume status, acute RV failure, pulmonary hypertension, prolonged ICU course

6. ± TEE probe

    (a) Caution with esophageal varices. May place TEE probe and not manipulate, leave in mid-esophageal 4 chamber view.

    (b) At least have available in room in case of emergency.

7. Airway

    (a) Largest size possible in case of fiberoptic bronchoscopy, pulmonary edema, suctioning

Preoperative Evaluation

1. Rapid sequence induction
   (a) All full-stomachs
   (b) Ascites
   (c) NPO status: called in from home, not planned
2. Hemodynamic state
   (a) Volume-depleted? Hemorrhaging?
3. Any contraindications to liver transplant?
   (a) Unstable arrhythmias
   (b) Severe pulmonary hypertension
4. Airway exam
   (a) Direct laryngoscopy ok?
   (b) Difficult intubation anticipated? – awake FOB
5. Cardiac function
   (a) Affects type of induction: any variation of etomidate, propofol with narcotic, benzodiazepines
6. Esophageal varices
   (a) Risk of TEE probe causing trauma, bleeding
7. Neurologic: mentation, hepatic encephalopathy
   (a) Hyperalgesia
8. Hematologic: coagulopathic? Prothrombotic? Thrombocytopenic?

Manifestations of Liver Disease and Their Anesthetic Implications

Adelmann et al. [1] (Table 40.2)

1. Neurological
   (a) Hepatic encephalopathy, coma, altered mental status, seizures, asterixis
   (b) In fulminant liver failure --> cerebral edema --> increased intracranial pressure --> herniation, intracerebral hemorrhage
   (c) Most liver failure patients will die of ICH
2. Cardiovascular
   (a) Hyperdynamic heart, high ejection fraction, low systemic vascular resistance, and high cardiac output.
   (b) If the liver disease is due to Wilson's disease which causes a cardiomyopathy, a low ejection fraction can be done.
3. Pulmonary
   (a) Restrictive lung physiology, decreased functional residual capacity due to ascites
   (b) Pulmonary edema, pleural effusions R > L

Table 40.2   Description of key events that occur during the pre-anhepatic, anhepatic, and reperfusion stages of a liver transplant

Phase	Event	Impact
Pre-anhepatic	Abdomen opened Ascites released Loss of tamponade effect on splanchnic vessels	Release ascites Improvement in functional residual capacity (FRC) and lung compliance Hemodynamic changes (hypotension, bradycardia)
	Usually coagulopathic	Surgeon may request pre-emptive fresh frozen plasma (FFP) and platelet transfusion to decrease bleeding during dissection
	Adhesions/scar tissue Portal hypertension Engorged splanchnic vessels	Difficult dissection High risk of traumatic injury to liver or blood vessels with hemorrhage May pre-emptively start pressors or give blood products Check ABG/TEG q20min minimum Keep volume low (low CVP) to decrease IVC distension and improve surgical view
	Lifting of liver	Loss of preload and therefore cardiac output Anticipate by watching surgeons carefully and giving pressors
	Acute vs. chronic liver failure	Acute liver failure: no time for collaterals; volume depleted Chronic liver failure: lots of collaterals
Anhepatic	Clamp vessels	Thrombus formation in IVC Significant drop in preload
	Anhepatic: no liver to make clotting factors or clear toxins	Massive bleeding potential, very high EBL Acidosis: give bicarbonate Coagulopathy: give blood products Frequent ABG/TEG q20min Glucose: hypoglycemia Hypocalcemia: massive transfusion; high citrate leading to calcium chelation Hyperkalemia: hyperventilation, bicarbonate Vasoplegia: loss of arterial waveform, hypotension Cold: Bair hugger on, warmed room; cold temperature worsens coagulopathy
	Waiting for surgeons to anastomose new liver	Organize your workstation Have a couple syringes of epinephrine, bicarbonate, and calcium setup Dilute epinephrine 10 mcg/ml in line ready to bolus Carefully watch TEE, EKG, and arterial lines

Table 40.2 (continued)

Phase	Event	Impact
Reperfusion	Cold, acidotic, hyperkalemic, high lactate, and high citrate blood is reperfused and recirculated Staged reperfusion: surgeons slowly unclamp	This is when bad things happen (cardiac arrest, acute RV failure, MI, etc.) Hypocalcemia → hypotension Hyperkalemia → arrhythmias Cold → arrhythmias, coagulopathy Massive blood loss → coagulopathy Acidosis → arrhythmias, myocardial ischemia/infarction, coagulopathy, hypotension Thrombi → arrhythmias, hypotension, pulmonary hypertension

4. Gastrointestinal
   (a) Ascites, esophageal varices, peptic ulcer disease
   (b) High aspiration risk because ascites, so do rapid sequence induction
   (c) Massive splanchnic vasodilation
5. Renal
   (a) Massive splanchnic vasodilation --> low renal perfusion pressure --> renal vascular urge tries to vasoconstrict by activating the renin-angiotensin-aldosterone system --> salt and water retention
   (b) Diagnosis of exclusion
   (c) Kidneys sense they are underperfused
6. Hematologic
   (a) Hypercoagulable and hypocoagulable
   (b) Even with an elevated INR, a patient's TEG can show hypercoagulability
   (c) Just because a patient has a high INR doesn't mean they have a propensity to bleed, because the INR tests for specific factors only
   (d) Liver makes factors 2, 7, 9, and 10, and proteins C and S, but proteins C and S have shorter half-lives
7. Endocrine
   (a) Impaired glucose homeostasis, decreased gluconeogenesis --> hypoglycemia
8. Infectious Disease
   (a) Prone to infection, bacterial translocation across gut wall
   (b) Everyone always thinks of spontaneous bacterial peritonitis, but the most common infection is actually pneumonia
9. Metabolic
   (a) Electrolyte imbalances, malnourished, chronically hyponatremic (water > sodium), hypokalemia, hypomagnesemia

(b) High volume of distribution – theoretically need higher dosage of induction drugs, but impaired hepatic metabolism of drug, so lasts longer, don't need higher doses in real life
10. Hepatorenal (see above)
11. Hepatopulmonary
    (a) Increased shunting from arterial to venous (right to left) within the intrapulmonary vasculature --> hypoxia
    (b) Do better when lie down because less shunting
    (c) Basically the liver makes and clears VEGF (vascular endothelial growth factor), and in liver failure, VEGF makes it to the pulmonary circulation and creates AVMs
12. Portopulmonary
    (a) Pulmonary hypertension due to portal hypertension (portal to systemic circulation)
    (b) Toxic mediators are not cleared by the failing liver --> systemic circulation --> severe pulmonary artery hypertension

Phases of Liver Transplant

Guidelines for Acute Massive Blood Loss (Table 40.3)

Table 40.3 Management of massive blood loss

Goal	Intervention	Comments
Call for help	Blood Bank OR RN OR Runner Massive Transfusion Protocol	Blood bank mobilizes 45 U packed red blood cells (PRBC), 45 U fresh frozen plasma (FFP), 4–6 U Platelets as soon as possible (ASAP) Blood bank supplies batches of 10 U PRBC, 10 U FFP, 1–2 U plt
Restore Volume	Large bore IV access, Central Line	
	Crystalloid, colloid	Caution w/dilutional anemia Caution w/coagulopathy Monitor CVP
	Blood products	Blood loss is often underestimated Caution w/coagulopathy Caution w/hypothermia Caution w/hypocalcemia
	Maintain normal BP and urine output (UOP)	Pressors, inotropes
Arrest bleeding	Early surgical intervention	
Monitor Labs	CBC, Coags, Fibrinogen, TEG ABG, BMP	

Contents of Blood Products

Blood products are separated into specific components which should be transfused according to the patient's coagulopathy status (Fig. 40.1 and Table 40.4)

- Cryo = factor VIII, factor XIII, vWF, fibrinogen
- 1 unit of FFP = 2 × fibrinogen and 2 × factor VIII in 1 unit of Cryoprecipitate
- 1 pack Cryo = 5 units Cryo
- Typical ratios of transfusion: 2–3: 2–3: 1 of PRBC: FFP: Plt

Fig. 40.1 Diagram outlining how whole blood is separated into individual components for blood transfusion

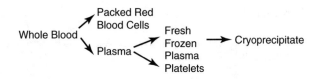

Table 40.4 Options for blood transfusion

Blood product	Special preparation	When to transfuse	How much to transfuse	Expected change
PRBCs	Fresh: <7 days old Washed if patient <1 year old or <10 kg	Hb < 7 Hct < 21 Clinically indicated	10–15 cc/kg	Increases Hb 2–3/Hct 6–9
FFP		½ × blood volume has been replaced w/PRBCs Excessive oozing without known cause	10–15 cc/kg	Increases factors 15–20%
Platelets		EBL > 1–2 × blood volumes Platelet count <100 K w/ further blood loss anticipated	5–10 cc/kg	Increases platelet count 50–100 K
Cryoprecipitate		Extensive blood loss replaced w/PRBC and FFP Clinical/laboratory evidence of coagulopathy Hypofibrinogenemia	5–10 cc/kg	Increases fibrinogen 60–100 mg/dL
Whole blood	<7 days old			Replace blood loss "cc per cc"
Reconstituted blood	Mix donor-matched PRBCs and FFP Irradiated Washed if >7 days old			Replace blood loss "cc per cc"

Non-blood Products
- Recombinant factors
- VIII, IX, VIIa, etc.
- K-Centra = PCC = Prothrombin Complex Concentrate = II, VII, IX, X, Protein C + S
- Antifibrinolytics
  - TXA = tranexaminic acid
  - Amicar = aminocaproic acid
- Protamine

Reference

1. Adelmann D, Kronish K, Ramsay MA. Anesthesia for liver transplantation. Anesthesiol Clin. 2017;35:491–508.

Index

© The Author(s), under exclusive license to Springer Nature Switzerland AG 2021
C. Sampankanpanich Soria et al., *Anesthesiology Resident Manual of Procedures*,
https://doi.org/10.1007/978-3-030-65732-1

Printed in the United States
by Baker & Taylor Publisher Services